CW00954246

Enlightened Weight Loss

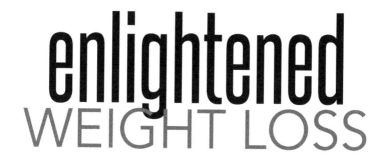

enlightened
WEIGHT LOSS

Breaking Free from The Inner Trap
of Endless Dieting

LINDA EVANS

NEW YORK

LONDON • NASHVILLE • MELBOURNE • VANCOUVER

enlightened WEIGHT LOSS

Breaking Free from The Inner Trap of Endless Dieting

© 2019 Linda Evans

All rights reserved. No portion of this book may be reproduced, stored in a retrieval system, or transmitted in any form or by any means—electronic, mechanical, photocopy, recording, scanning, or other—except for brief quotations in critical reviews or articles, without the prior written permission of the publisher.

Published in New York, New York, by Morgan James Publishing in partnership with Difference Press. Morgan James is a trademark of Morgan James, LLC. www.MorganJamesPublishing.com

ISBN 9781642792126 paperback
ISBN 9781642792133 eBook
Library of Congress Control Number: 2018908637

Cover Design by:
Megan Dillon
megan@creativeninjadesigns.com

Interior Design by:
Chris Treccani
www.3dogcreative.net

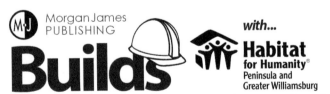

Morgan James is a proud partner of Habitat for Humanity Peninsula and Greater Williamsburg. Partners in building since 2006.

Get involved today! Visit
MorganJamesPublishing.com/giving-back

*For my sister Barbara, whose Light infuses my
life and all of the pages of this book.*

Table of Contents

Introduction   *ix*

Chapter 1   Diets and Addictions   1
Chapter 2   Self-Awareness   19
Chapter 3   Inner Detective   31
Chapter 4   Feel to Heal   47
Chapter 5   Own Your Behaviors   59
Chapter 6   Be Kind   71
Chapter 7   Enlightened Living   83
Chapter 8   Supportive Resources   95
Chapter 9   The Journey Continues   105
Chapter 10   Conclusion   117

Further Reading   *123*
Acknowledgments   *125*
About the Author   *129*
Thank You   *131*

Introduction

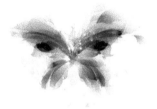

*"Out beyond ideas of wrongdoing and
rightdoing, there is a field. I'll meet you there."*
– RUMI

You Are Not Alone in Your Dieting Woes
and
It's Not Your Fault

Have you spent the majority of your life with the feeling, "I need to lose weight!"?

Are you hoping to leave a different legacy for your children?

If so, this book is for you.

If you're like me, and the majority of people I've known in my life, this might be a very familiar scenario to you: A new diet finds its way to you that looks like it has potential to help you shed the pounds you've put on since the last time you dieted. You're skeptical, but upon closer examination, you see it incorporating all of the best bits of the past diets you've been on that have worked for you. It is a more balanced eating plan – one you feel you would be able to follow and maintain for life!

You have a hard time getting started on it, but since this isn't your first go-round in the dieting rodeo, within the first two weeks, you find yourself adjusting to this new way of eating. You have more energy and see the pounds rolling off! Within a few months, you've lost the original weight you wanted to and more, and you are feeling great! Your hopes are up that this could very well be the eating plan you have been waiting for – and the one that you and your family can stick to for life.

Things are going well, and you enjoy a nice vacation with the family, you have more energy to take on that extra project at work, and you agree to volunteer in a new way at your child's school. Life is great! You are super busy and come home tired most nights, and have less time to cook, so the family eats out more and more. One day you wake up and feel your pants are much tighter than they've been in a while and you can't button them up. You realize your energy has been low again for quite a while, and you realize you've been eating "off plan" again. But now you're so tired that you just don't feel like continuing to eat the way you know you should, and you don't have the energy to even make the effort if you did want to. Within a few weeks, your lost pounds, along with some added friends, are back on your body and you're wondering how you got back to this place – again!

If this sounds like you, the most important thing to become aware of is that you're not alone. Not only is the above scenario one I myself am intimately familiar with, I've also worked with countless other fellow human journeyers who have had the same dilemma over the course of my years as a self-awareness coach and mentor.

And let's face it. If a diet or an eating plan exists that would have gotten you over the weight-loss finish line by now, you would have found it. You're smart, you're able to start and stick to diets (at least for a time), and you could have written a dissertation on the topic of diet and exercise at this point in the game. But life always seems to get in the way and derail your best efforts, every time. You're not alone, and if you're like me, you've not only seen these dramas at play within your own life, but probably also within the lives of your family and friends.

I've come to see that this is no longer just a personal issue – it has become an epidemic. In fact, there are enough of us looking to lose weight (again ... and again ... and again!) that the dieting and weight-loss industry is about a $60 billion industry in the US alone! The convincing tale we are sold is that, if we would just follow this diet to a tee, take that supplement, or adopt the latest watcha-ma-whozits eating plan, all would be well. And yet with an estimated 45 million Americans going on a diet each year, and spending $33 billion each year on weight loss products, nearly two-thirds of Americans are still overweight or obese.

Obviously, something else must be going on beneath the surface of diets, rules, and fads that proclaim there is one right or best way for all humans to eat and exercise to be forever thin and healthy. If that were the case, and it were that easy – to simply be told: "Here are the foods you should eat and this is how you should exercise, and you'll reach and forever maintain your ideal weight," and you would magically be able to *pull that off*, you would have done it by now. *And* if we all could do that, it would be the end of the diet industry.

What *would not* keep the diet industry in place would be a planet full of people at peace within themselves, particularly with regard to their weight. It is kept in place by marketers convincing us all that having a thin, buff body is going to be the only way to get love, to fit in (and to rule the world!). The narrative is: "If you could just lose weight, you'd have it all!" And as icing on the proverbial cake, the food industry aids and abets the weight-loss industry by pushing its cheaper-to-manufacture sugary and refined foods on us at every turn.

Now don't get me wrong. There *is* a place in our lives for this type of awareness, and we can gain a lot of benefits from the food and nutrition information to be found out on the web and in bookstores. I have benefitted in many ways over the years from adjusting my eating: from eating low-carb/high-protein, to cutting out all sugars and refined flours, to juice cleansing, to food combining, and intermittent fasting. All of these plans were good for me at the time, but none of them were a final solution to my weight issues. This is because, as I came to find out, my weight issues had less to do with the food I was putting into my body and more to do with *how I was feeling* any time I put that food into my body.

In this book, I will be inviting you to go on a journey with me, to a place and a time in your life when you lived happy and free – before your dieting stories began. Deep within the heart of you, you will find a little-child-*you* who is still alive – living and breathing and waiting for you to look to *her* once again with love – no matter how much she weighs, and no matter what she is doing. Only by spending this sort of quality time with her are you going to get to the *heart* of your weight-loss issues.

If you're intrigued, I invite you to read on, playful and curious like a child. These two characteristics of small children bring magic and wonder to the world. And they are the same characteristics on which the magic of your future journey to your perfectly-weighted self rides.

In writing this book, and taking a look back at my life, it became clear to me that I've spent the majority of my life either in the process of losing weight or having to be vigilant at keeping off my newly lost pounds. Whenever I did lose weight, I was happy that I'd lost the weight, but I knew I'd have to be careful not to "slip" into my old patterns and gain the weight back. Other times, when looking into mirrors, even at what would be considered an "ideal" weight, I would usually at some point watch my thoughts float over to thinking about how I could make some portion of my body better – more attractive, healthier, or more toned.

Does this sound familiar? Over the years, through all of these phases, I've often felt alone in my struggle, as if the stories around my own weight issues were vastly different to the ones other people faced; as if my relationship to eating and to my body was somehow a secret shame I shouldn't mention to others, because I didn't want to admit I was in that struggle. Over the past 15 years, working with and hearing the stories of hundreds of women and men from all different walks of life, I've come to deeply understand that I'm not alone; and neither were they (*and neither are you!*). And while this has helped me, and them, get a kind of inner relief of sorts – knowing that we're not alone in our struggles – it has also brought up deep sadness within me, particularly as I watch children at younger and younger ages jump into the storyline of "My body has to be changed so I can be loved!"

In conversations with so many friends – women in particular – they have been sharing how this obsession with weight seems now to be even more all-pervasive, and a focus for their children at a much younger age than it even was for them.

I remember myself at 11 years old being a kid of average size, maybe a little pudgy, thinking I needed to find a way to lose weight, maybe by eating less every day. I thought it through and realized I didn't like mornings much anyway, so I said: "I wonder if I would lose weight if I were to skip breakfasts?" And I proceeded to skip breakfasts, and even sometimes sleep in so I would have less time in my day to worry about eating. And what was the reason I wanted to lose weight? So I could become as thin as the girls who seemed to be more popular in school and have more friends (in my little girl's eyes). I didn't think about the other aspects of my personality that might be playing a role in my "popularity" – like my shyness or my very different take on the world than theirs. I had somehow already learned to relate my "acceptability" factor to the shape of my body. And it's not that I was what one might call a shallow kid – focused only on external appearances and looks. I was a kid who did a lot of internal thinking and searching, a little philosopher and poet from a very early age and through grade school, and yet I didn't see this dynamic at play regarding my sudden desires to lose weight.

If you're with me so far, you're likely also taking a look back upon your own journey through your life so far with regard to your weight-loss stories and dramas. How much of your life has been taken up by thoughts of dieting, exercising, and needing to lose all that extra weight you gained? How often have you successfully dieted, finding a way of eating you thought would finally be the one way you'd be able to stick to for life, only to see yourself at some point come right back to – or well past – the weight you'd started at?

If you're ready to find a new way to step outside of these repeating patterns, read on. This book is not going to give you another set of rules about the best way to get you to lose weight and maintain that weight loss for life. I'm sure you will be able to find *plenty* of those books elsewhere if that's what you're looking for. Instead, this book is going to take you on a journey behind the scenes of the dieting hamster-wheel that you, I, and so many of our friends have been on; and upon which we have spun out of control every time. The goal of this book is to help you uncover what keeps tripping you up and what keeps you spinning your wheels year after year in this way. Only once you do that will any of the ways of eating you've explored up to now be able to impact your weight and your life positively forever.

It should be clear at this point that we are talking about an epidemic here. Not only because of the rise in obesity we see happening all around us, but even more so because there is such an *obsession* and *focus out there* for making ourselves wrong if we are not walking around in a body the world considers to be the "right size and shape." In this book, I'll also be inviting you to explore how and why it has come to pass – that even with so many of us having this obsession and focus on dieting and exercise routines to get us that right-sized body – we, as a nation, are heavier than we've ever been before. What is going on?

There are multiple things at play, not the least of which is the $60 billion diet industry's agenda to sell us more and more of its diet plans, health foods, and exercise regimes. When you add that together with the food-industry catering to our sugar and wheat addictions, it starts to become clear what we're up against. These two things alone actually put us at such a disadvantage, against a subtle giant of epic proportions, that it makes sense we would all be on this wheel and cycle of losing weight and then re-gaining that weight, only to have to lose it all again.

If you gain nothing else from this book but that by the end of it you are finally able to *cut yourself some slack* around your weight-loss issues, your time here will have been well spent! The stresses we put ourselves under, each and every time we imagine the worst about ourselves because of what bad food choices we have put into our bodies, are tremendous! Every time we cast ourselves into the unlovable bucket because of our body shape, we add another stress onto the heap. No wonder it's so hard to be at peace with our dieting when you consider this dynamic going on!

Imagine taking a very small child – maybe one who has a few extra pounds on her – and sending her out into this huge world of sugary treats, distracted eating, and stressful situations. Make sure she also sits in front of image after image of (Photoshopped) super-slim models and movie stars so she gets the message in her little subconscious that there's something wrong with her as she notices her body does not look like theirs. And finally, give her a set of rules about food and eating – *and exercise!* – that she'll have to always follow if she ever hopes to get (and keep) her body down to that acceptable size.

Would she have a chance at being at peace within herself around food, eating, and her body shape and size? Just imagine the overwhelm that beautiful little creature would experience!

Next imagine sitting down with her little self, after seeing how she isn't able to handle all that stress *and* follow the rules around eating and moving her body in the right ways you gave to her; and picture her struggling with all of the other 'shoulds' she hasn't been able to succeed at. She can't keep up and she feels like a failure and has begun to internalize the feeling that something is very wrong with her. Would you think she is a failure and a bad girl or would you see what she's up against? Now, imagine instead of comforting her and letting her know how beautiful she is, you instead start berating her. You let her know how bad she is because she ate way too much sugar today. Why did she eat those extra desserts? You yell at her because she didn't run enough on the playground, even though you know it's because she was trying to cope with all of the pressure and she needed some private time on the swings. You put her down because she didn't eat the healthy food you told her she had to eat.

Now put yourself in her shoes. Do you think dealing with her in this way will help her have an easier time of things tomorrow on the playground? Will it help her eat and live more healthily within her little life?

Hopefully you can see what a *weight* that treating her in this way would put on her little self and psyche. Expecting her to focus this hard on what she eats and does and how she looks would be a battle that would be impossible for her to win.

And yet, I'm willing to bet that at some point in your life, you have done something this horrible (or worse) to yourself on a daily basis with regard to your body, your weight, and your eating patterns. If you are berating yourself, pushing yourself, and focusing on the ways in which you were weak today with your eating or your exercising – in the hopes it'll motivate you to be better tomorrow – then you are putting yourself under exactly the same impossible stress and strain that the innocent little girl above wouldn't be able to win with.

If this is speaking to you, and you can relate to the incredible pressure you put yourself under when it comes to your weight and dieting issues, I invite you to use the above journey through your imagination to create for yourself a sense of greater empathy, and a little more understanding, with this clearer picture of what you're up against. With this book, my further hope for you is that this empathy will only continue to grow for you as you find new ways to conquer the weight-loss dramas you've been living through your whole life.

You are in good hands here. Firstly, know that you are not alone. Secondly, know that you are not some sort of crazed freak who just can't figure out how to pull together the willpower and inner strength and stick-to-itiveness you think – if you only had them – would get you everything you think you want with regard to your body and your weight. And finally, know that the first step in making any change is to first understand the problem, and then to face it head on. Through this book and the process outlined in it, you will discover a practical set of tools that will help you finally get to the heart of your weight-loss issues in a much more peaceful, gentle, and loving way.

This book is going to take you on a fun and healing journey within yourself, where you will meet your Inner Innocent; get assistance from your Inner Detective; be guided by your Inner Health Guru; and uncover your hidden Inner Bully and Inner Guard Dog. You will learn how to stop these energies within you from tripping you up in the future. The tools and techniques I'll be sharing have worked not only in my own life, but also in the lives of my many clients over the years, and I know they can also help get *you* to end the cycle of forever-dieting once and for all – with no self-flagellation whip required!

Within each chapter, you will find a step or technique, along with some practical tools to use to help you get off of the crazy cycles you have been stuck on throughout your weight-loss journey, step by gentle step. Your journey within is going to get you a better understanding of how to get off of this cycle of forever-dieting once and for all, no matter how many times before you have found yourself in these situations over the course of your life.

If this all sounds good to you, please read on, and settle into the knowing that this is going to be a gentle yet powerful journey; a journey that has the very real potential to change your life forever, from the inside out.

Chapter 1
Diets and Addictions

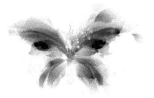

"Your task? To work with all the passion of your being to acquire an inner light."

– RUMI

Dieting and Addiction Dilemmas We All Face, and Why It's Time to Jump Ship and Swim in a New Direction

In the Introduction, you may have noticed that I mentioned the words sugar and addiction more than once when describing the dieting dilemmas we all face. This wasn't by accident. On my own journey through food obsession, enjoyment, restriction, and attempted-control, there are two substances that always in retrospect could be seen to have had an addictive hold over me anytime I would eat (or drink) them. One of them was sugar, and the other, coffee.

Throughout my exploration of eating plans and diets, cleanses, and fasts, I would find I would gain a clearer head and more focused brain as an added benefit to the weight I was losing anytime I was following one of the more restrictive eating plans. I would suddenly have the ability to focus more clearly, and sense an overall increase in my energy levels and my ability to maintain that energy over the course of the day. I always assumed this was because of my healthier weight and the loss of some of the toxins I had been accumulating through less-than-ideal food choices.

However, whenever I would then switch back to what (I always hoped) would be a maintenance way of eating, I would invariably find that my energy levels would sink back down, my brain would get foggy, and it would get harder for me to do my work efficiently. This shift from one state to the other was particularly extreme after the types of diets I was following that were cleanses or fasts of some sort.

In looking back on this, one culprit I noticed that would kick-start the low-energy and cycle of me wanting more of something to try to maintain my energy levels when I went back to "normal eating" was coffee. I discovered it wasn't the caffeine as such, but particularly the coffee that had this effect on me. So I decided (since I loved the taste of coffee), that I would go back to drinking it, but I would just have one cup of good coffee in the morning, and that should keep me from getting too worn out by it. But by mid-day I'd find myself tired, and the only thing I would want or be drawn to eat or drink would be another cup of coffee – in order to pick myself back up (I would tell myself). It turns out (I would see in hindsight), that the extra coffee never *would* pick me back up, but would actually instead drop my energy and decrease my brain focus – and not too long after drinking it would then – you guessed it – make me want to grab another cup of coffee!

You might be thinking, "Isn't this normal, and how all of us are throughout the day and with coffee in particular? Isn't this one of the benefits of coffee?" Well, I can tell you that for my own life, when I discovered what was going on, and I took the (painful) action of cutting out coffee completely again from my life, my energy levels returned, such that I no longer craved, or needed, *any* coffee. After I discovered this dynamic, I decided that *for me,* I had to treat coffee drinking in particular as a full-on addiction. I wouldn't say that everyone has this same addiction (because no two bodies are exactly alike), but for me personally, over the course of *many* years, I finally came to understand this. And I learned that when I'm not drinking coffee, I feel more energized, and I don't miss it at all!

At one point recently, however, after doing quite a bit of amazing inner, energetic work that had gotten my body feeling particularly healthy and resilient, I told myself I should be able to enjoy all things in moderation, without having to feel any sense of restriction with anything – as I'd come to experience with food items (more on that to come). So it came to be that one day, as I smelled someone's coffee, and remembered how yummy it can be to have at the end of a good meal, I decided to enjoy a cup. And I did enjoy it fully.

The next day, I found myself going out to buy some good coffee beans – to have on occasion (I told myself). And then I bought a single-serve coffee press (since I no longer had any coffee-making equipment). And oh, I told myself – I better also get that awesome burr grinder. Once I had all of that, I decided I should then at least make one cup of good coffee a day to enjoy. After a few days, after a particularly long morning, when break time came around, I decided that because the coffee smelled so good, and it seemed to no longer really be affecting me as it used to, I would have another cup. Later that same day, I went for another cup. And before I knew it, I was drinking several coffees a day again, every day. And I was suddenly back onto the cycle of my coffee drinking addiction.

I write all this *not* to say that coffee is bad for me, or for you, or for anyone else. I'm writing this to show the insidious way in which addictions work and affect us – and how they can, and do, work their way into, out of, and then back into our lives again – usually without us ever even really being aware of this dynamic being at play.

Before I continue, it may be good to explore the word addiction a bit more, particularly for the purposes of this book, which is about your (and humanity's) weight-loss woes, so you can see exactly what you've been up against as you've tried to get a handle on your food choices and various eating patterns as you've been scampering along over the years on your weight-loss hamster wheel.

To be addicted to something is to be physically and mentally dependent on a particular substance and unable to stop taking it without incurring adverse effects. It can also mean: to be enthusiastically devoted to a particular thing or activity; obsessed with; devoted to; fixated on; fanatical about; enamored; dependent.

I don't know about you, but these definitions describe both my relationship to most foods (especially the ones I "know" aren't good for me: sugary, fatty, and fried foods) as well as my obsession with food in general – watching what I eat; buying organic; eating a healthy balance of carbs, protein, fiber, and fat; getting all of the right supplements; etc.

I can say that I've been both obsessed with the foods I know I "shouldn't" eat as well as the foods I love eating. Can you relate? I've also noticed I feel a distinct sense of having to sacrifice my joy in life if I try (or feel I have to try) to go without these favorite foods of mine for any length of time.

So.... Would this be considered an addiction? It does fit the description given above to me. It is something for you to explore and look at more closely in your own life as you step upon this *ENLIGHTENED Weight Loss* journey and discover with new eyes where you've been and where you're going, with regard to having a healthy body and a healthy relationship to your body and to the food you put in it.

The word *addiction* is usually used to describe a dependency on substances other than the very things we need to keep our bodies functioning – substances like alcohol, cocaine, or heroin. For the purposes of this book, I invite you to consider where in your life the quality of *addictive dependency* may have come into play in your life with regard to the *foods* you have eaten or in terms of your eating and dieting patterns – now, and over the years.

Please, please, please tread lightly here. When you look back, please look with compassionate, neutral eyes on every observation from your past. It will be best to look back with the eyes of a detective, who is looking on a crime-scene of sorts to discover clues that might help to solve this particularly puzzling case at hand. It won't serve you to judge the past behaviors if your goal is to learn something new about your eating patterns so you can rewrite your weight-loss story. The act of judging will take this Inner Detective of yours right out of his flow.

So as you look back, consider if you have ever found one or two foods that for you, at different times of eating them, would fall into the addictive category for you? Look back in your life for those areas that might point to addiction, like binging when alone; *having* to always eat dessert after dinner; not being able to resist sweets if they're sitting out at a party or offered to you; craving salty snacks after a stressful day; etc. Are the foods you ate during these times ones that would fall into the category of foods for which you know you become out-of-control physiologically or mentally? Ones on which you feel dependent and unable to stop eating without adverse effects? If so, this gives you a clue, that what you're up against is not "just" your willpower. When there is an addiction, there are actual physiological and emotional components at play that can and do trip you up. This means that, around these foods, no matter what heroic efforts you might put into your intake of them, you are fighting against a physiological dynamic that is stronger than you might realize.

For instance, studies have shown that refined sugar is a more addictive substance than cocaine. Interestingly, refined sugar is a white crystal extracted from a plant (sugar cane), just as cocaine is a white crystal extracted from a plant (coca leaves). Eating coca leaves is not addictive, nor does it have the same effects on the body as ingesting cocaine does. The same has been found to be true with sugar. Natural and raw sugar cane does not produce an addictive response, but when the sugar is extracted from the sugar cane and made into a refined powder, its molecular structure is changed, and the refined sugar can be highly addictive. Sugar can be so addictive that, in animal studies, poor rats who researchers had gotten hooked on cocaine through IVs almost all switched over to sugar once it was introduced to them.

So OK, just like my addiction to coffee, you may say that you can take sweets or leave them. And so *you* may not be afflicted by this curse that so many of us others are. Before you finalize that conclusion, however, I invite you to also look at all of the packaged and prepared foods you may eat or crave throughout the day, including even the dressings you may like to smother your healthy salad in, or the lattes or sodas you add into your days at regular intervals.

Again, I am not saying all of this in order to try to introduce a new diet plan to you that will get you unhooked from sugar (although there are great ones out there that do have suggestions for helping you do just that, most notably for me: *Bright Line Eating* by Susan Peirce Thompson). I simply want to bring your attention to this as a challenging aspect of your dieting woes – that you might not always look at so consciously – so you are better able to appreciate the physiological and mental components that are also at play. This can help you uncouple your eating struggles from your sense of not having enough *willpower;* or from you feeling you're not "disciplined enough" when you aren't able to break some of these addictive patterns. I hope this might also put into perspective the pointless nature of the harsh attacks you so often receive from yourself – from what I am going to call your Inner Bully (more about her in a bit).

There have been other studies exploring addictions, which look at why some people may be more susceptible to various addictions than others. For instance, some people are exposed to addictive opiate painkillers during surgeries and are able to keep from getting addicted to them while others cannot. While there is likely a physiological reason for this – where some people are more physiologically susceptible than others – there have also been studies done with rats which suggest a different possible explanation. In what was called the "Rat Park" experiment, it was found that rats who were not isolated, but rather who were able to be in a community of other rats, were *much* more able to walk away from addictive substances than the ones who were kept isolated.

This is why Johann Hari, in his book *Chasing the Scream: The First and Last Days of the War on Drugs,* wrote: "For a hundred years now we've been singing war songs about addicts. I think all along we should have been singing love songs to them. Because the opposite of addiction is not sobriety; the opposite of addiction is connection."

My invitation to you as we explore where within this addiction spectrum you may be, is that you start singing love songs to yourself instead of war songs. The guidelines, tools, and steps in this book are going to be used to help guide you along this path of *self-gentleness* and *self-compassion*, using a step-by-step process I call the ENLIGHTEN Process. With it, you will not only work on lightening your body, but even more importantly, you'll begin being able to truly *enlighten* yourself, from the inside out. This means shedding a light on the harsh task-master actions your Inner Weight-Loss Bully has been directing your way all of these years. Another way you'll be able to get an enlightened sense of yourself will be by removing the *weight* of all of the stresses you've been attaching, without self-compassion, to your whole weight-loss dilemma for so much of your life.

And while we are on the topic of addictions, I'd like to bring to your awareness another addiction you may not have thought about as an addiction. This is an addiction I've found to be way more pervasive than any food or substance addiction – in that I've seen it in *all* the humans I've worked with. I call this addiction I've seen an addiction to our *"selves."* It's an addiction to the sense of ourselves we think of as "me" or "who I am"; to the learned set of behaviors that guide our actions and define us. This sense of self is actually made up of patterns and behaviors we learned and took on as we were growing up – and it has become who we think we *are*. More importantly, we have learned that we must stick to this way of being in order to stay safe out in the world around us. Another more common expression for this sense of self and the patterns and habits of living we have become addicted to would be: our *comfort zone*.

There are many names we can and do give to these patterns, behaviors and thoughts that define us:

- My self (ego-based sense of "who I am")
- My identity (the set of qualities that make me uniquely "me")
- My comfort zone (the place I know it's safe to stay in because I've lived from it my whole life – even though it may no longer be serving me to stay there)
- My belief systems (the rules for living I've learned from my culture, my family, and my environment)
- My blocks (the places my belief systems trip me up whenever I want to do something that differs from those things I learned were "safe" to want or to get)
- My hang-ups (the patterns I see repeating over and over again in my life even though I know better)

For all of the above, I like to simply say these all represent who we think we are, and who we have learned we *have* to be in order to keep up our identity – our sense of self. They also represent how we have learned we need to behave and act in order to be loved, to fit in, to be accepted, and to "make it" in the world. When you consider that the number one need of a human being is safety, then it's not a far stretch to see that our need to stay within these patterns or rules-for-safety we learned becomes all-important to us, especially in our formative years, just as we are trying to navigate the world of "the scary big people" around us. This means that the majority of these beliefs about "who we are" get put into place in our most formative years – from the ages of 0 to 4 years old.

Since these rules about how we had to live to fit in and be safe in our environment were so important to us, they necessarily had to become things we could *depend* on staying consistently in place inside of us. In order for this to happen, a need or *dependency* got set up, in the realm below our conscious mind, such that we would be sure to follow these "rules for our safety" at all times. And as we've seen, another word for having a dependency on something, without which we would suffer adverse effects, is: an *addiction.*

So we can say that a pattern of *addiction* was set up within us – an addiction to *self*, an addiction to *who we need to be;* an addiction to not rocking the boat; an addiction to staying the same; an addiction to the status quo; an addiction to not learning or making lasting changes if they were to go counter to our previously established rules for safety.

There are many books, self-help programs, and 12-step programs available for us to deal with our various addictions to substances, from alcohol to drugs to food. And for sure, these are and can be great tools to help you beat any of these types of addictions you might have. They provide participants with a supportive team of people who are there to get you out of the isolation game of your particular addiction and into a community of connection.

But rarely do these programs directly address the addiction we all have to our *self*, which is to say to our belief systems, patterns of behavior, and "rules for safety" that keep tripping us up mentally and emotionally whenever we start to make new conscious changes in our lives, particularly if those changes go against the old rules we learned for "who we are" which are safely tucked away beyond our conscious knowledge of them. These are the limiting beliefs we learned as our "truth" – because they at some point served the purpose of keeping us safe.

Examples of some of these rules are:

"I'll never be able to get it all together to take care of myself."

"If I lose weight, I'll get too much attention from men who will want me for one reason only."

"I am incapable of success. Why even try?"

"Who am I to be great?"

"I have no willpower!"

Or, maybe you have rules more along these lines:

"You are so smart and strong – you should be able to get that weight off and keep it off – what's *wrong* with you?"

"If you can't get control of your weight, it shows just how lazy and weak-willed you are." And so on, and so on.

Some of these are the voices of what I earlier called your Inner Bully. Others are aspects of what I like to call your Inner Guard Dog. To understand what I mean by your Inner Guard Dog, imagine there is a loving, protective, and loyal guard dog who lives within you just like a beloved pet. She keeps you company and has been your lifelong companion, and it is her job to protect you from danger. She is the aspect of you whose job it has been to keep you safely following your beliefs about yourself and about *who you learned you need to be* in order to keep you safely tucked into your previously learned set of patterns and habits. And just like a loving guard dog in your home, your Inner Guard Dog would never try to intentionally hurt you. If you find her keeping you addicted to your old patterns and ways of being, know that is her way of trying to protect you. She isn't barking out negative statements and limiting rules just to be mean or to keep you down. She only barks these limiting rules out to you if they are ones you learned you needed to hold onto in order to safely navigate the world around you. Your Inner Guard Dog's real job has been to *protect* you, in the best way she learned how to – by making sure you never strayed far from the *you* that you learned you needed to be. This was meant to keep you from doing anything outside of your known zone of safety that has dictated who you need to be in order to stay safe in your world.

If you look at this in terms of your goals to lose weight and keep it off, you might find there are beliefs you learned in order to keep yourself safe that might be in direct opposition to conscious beliefs and desires you now have for your weight and your life. If getting what you consciously want would go against a previously learned rule, the older rule, because it was imprinted in your unconscious for your safety, will always win out – until you see it for what it is. For example, if you learned, "It's not safe to show my true self to the world," or "I have to hide my true self in order to not get hurt," then doing something that would allow you to shine – like becoming your ideal weight and dressing like you've always wanted to – would be seen as unsafe, because it would "show your true self." And so your Inner Guard Dog would find a way to sabotage you and your efforts, and perhaps even find ways to make you gain weight again (for instance).

If this is sounding complicated, take a breath, relax your shoulders, and tune into your inner world for a moment. Rest assured that this will make more and more sense to you as we go. For now, see if you can feel your Inner Guard Dog. She is that aspect of your brain whose job it is to manage your activities in order to keep you on the safe course of following the rules you learned you needed in order to make it in the world   as your small-self *you*. Are her ears up? Is she on high alert? Perhaps she is sensing you're on to her tricks. Maybe she's sending out the signal to you right now that this is all too confusing and complicated, in the hopes she can divert your attention and keep your Inner Detective (who you will meet in the next chapter) from following new inner clues that have been introduced here. Who knows? It is this mystery we will be unraveling together. I promise you, it is not complicated. And I will be guiding you step by step along the way, giving you the tools you'll need as you go. These will act as tasty morsels of meat for your Inner Guard Dog, so that even she will soon see that it's a new day and the world is safer out there than it was when she learned the tricks to keep you safe following that outdated set of rules. Soon she will be trotting alongside you as your happy companion on your journey to inner weight-loss enlightenment.

In the upcoming chapters, you will be exploring ways of working with your Inner Guard Dog; you will be able to meet her where she's coming from; and you'll be able to use her strong will, determination, and grit to start working in your favor on the new patterns of living you'd like to adopt – the ones you know would be healthier for you at this adult stage of your life – instead of keeping you within your child state of fear, lack, weakness of will, self-sabotage, etc.

Simply understanding these dynamics that are at play, and using such playful, simple imagery, goes a long way toward making the process a gentle and straightforward one as you move along into your brave new world of loving your body, your life, your actions, and your *Self*.

The ENLIGHTEN step-by-step process will help you take these steps into new territories, as you test out the waters of the realm outside of your comfort zone in a more conscious way. In this way, you will be able to determine with your adult senses if it's indeed a scary world out there, or if it is now the safer, happier, more loving, and dieting-free land of freedom you've been envisioning for yourself, and maybe even more importantly, for your family.

After exploring and coming into this new relationship with your outdated belief systems during the ENGLIGHTEN Process, you'll be pleasantly surprised to find another side-effect available to you: you will also be *lightening up* the amount of constant stress you've been under because of your constant self-berating inner dialog. And *this* is a side-effect you can truly *live* with, as it will give you another powerful

Inner Ally to support you to becoming the healthiest and happiest version of yourself.

There is a lot of research showing the link between the stress-hormone cortisol – which gets released during times of stress – and over-eating and weight-gain. During tension-filled times (which are constant if you are always beating yourself up for not "eating like you know you should,") the stress hormone, *cortisol*, rises and creates higher insulin levels. These higher insulin levels then drop your blood sugar, causing you to crave sugary and fatty foods. And so you then eat them, and then berate yourself for doing so. This in turn creates even *more* stress within you – and a vicious cycle ensues. Well isn't that just lovely?! This is another one of those traps that your Inner Guard Dog has been able to use to keep you within your old comfort zone of outdated beliefs. The negative attacks on yourself bring on stress, which releases more cortisol, which then keeps you from making any new, lasting change.

Another factor I'd like to call your attention to – as an added benefit of following the steps and principles of the ENLIGHTEN Process – is a benefit you will gain in relation to your sleep patterns. With the added physical and mental stress that beating yourself up for these actions has created in you, it's likely also true that sleeping and getting the right amount of sleep has become that much more difficult. And guess what? Not getting enough sleep can *also* contribute to weight-gain and out-of-control cravings around food. Some studies even suggest that if you get too little sleep, you are likely to gain up to nine times as much weight as you would if you had a full night's sleep on a regular basis. Yowzers!

Lastly, you will be taking steps to learn and explore a gentler path toward change than the one you've been on until now. You will be *unlearning* the patterns that no longer serve you, which means you will also be getting what I call an *enlightened sense of being*, because your stress load will be lessened tremendously, as well. As a final added bonus, you'll also be gaining a few new friends along the way (your Inner Detective, your Inner Guard Dog, and your Inner Innocent, to name just a few).

If this sounds intriguing to you, then get ready to take your first steps upon this path that will help you stop the mad cycle of self-berating and self-hate you've been on with regard to your eating patterns and your weight. Not only has your old negative self-talk *not* been helping you lose the weight you know you could be losing, it's been making your journey just downright unpleasant! These conflicting patterns within you – the old unconscious ones that have a hold on you without you knowing it, and the new conscious ones you want for yourself – are what are at the heart of your eating and dieting traumas and dilemmas to date. Fighting this internal struggle also has a huge impact on your energy levels, your inner-peace levels, and your ability-to-be-a-happy-human levels, far beyond your weight, and far beyond what you may have ever imagined.

Chapter 2

Self-Awareness

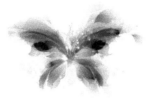

"Maybe you are searching among the branches,
for what only appears in the roots."

– RUMI

Self-Awareness Is the Key to Rewriting Your Weight Loss Story

Step 1: Engage Your Inner Witness – Look Within with Curious Eyes

For the purposes of this book and this process, the word *story*, as I talk about *Rewriting Your Weight-Loss Story,* is meant to represent the "fictional narrative of the weight-loss incidents and events of your life." Sure, there *is* a "factual" set of incidents and events you could *say* describes your life as you look back on it, and back on the journey you've been on as you've struggled to get control of your weight. However, in this chapter the assumption you will be making, as you take a look back at the past events of your life with new eyes, is that some of these past stories have been a kind of trance-inducing fiction that was made up when you were very young in order to keep you safe.

To help get you out of this trance, you will be using Step 1 of the ENLIGHTEN Process to first engage your Inner Witness, who will help you look within with curious eyes at your past behaviors, patterns, habits, and weight-loss and body image stories to see if they really do define *who you are,* or if they can be seen to fit into the category of "old rules for safety." You will enlist the help of your neutral, and very observant, Inner Detective to look upon the events in your life not only with a curiosity for how they have been affecting you, but also to see how they would look to you if they were things happening to your closest friend.

From this new perspective, you may see that what you've always considered as the "facts" of your journey were, in actual fact, influenced instead by that wily character introduced in the last chapter: your Inner Guard Dog. Remember, she is the one who's been trying, out of love and protection, to keep you tied blindly to your set of old and potentially outdated rules. It could be that she has also been pulling the wool over your eyes all these years in terms of how you've been seeing your life events. This means it likely is going to take some patience and inner compassion, together with some humble querying, to get to the true heart of the matter.

Step 1 of the ENGLIGHTEN Process is deceivingly simple: all you are going to do is *Engage Your Inner Witness and Look Within with Curious Eyes.* You will be exploring the issues that come up for you with regard to your weight and dieting issues from different angles, in order to start the process of becoming your own detective. You'll be looking at *the clues* of what has really been going on for you throughout the story of your ups and downs on your weight-loss roller coaster. This portion of the process is the foundation for the work to come, so it's important to really take the time to honor this step and to drop down into yourself as fully as possible. You might want to grab a journal or a notebook and have it handy as you read through the book and begin your ENLIGHTEN journey so you can jot down any notes or insights as they come up for you.

Right now, start by simply noticing, without judgment or the need to adjust anything, the current feeling/sensing state of your body. How deeply or shallowly are you breathing? What is the level of tension in your shoulders? Your hips? Your belly? Can you feel *all* of your body, or are there places that aren't "registering"? Are there parts of your body that you notice stand out and bother you more than others? Can you sense your feet? Are you aware of the pressure of the seat or the surface you are sitting or resting on?

Your job at this point of the process is simply to observe and take notice of all that you are sensing and feeling. Let any thoughts or feelings about your various body parts as you do this exercise simply arise. If any thoughts surface which seem significant or don't seem to want to go away, take those as your prompt that something to look at has come up. Jot it down on your notepad, and write a summary of what came up for you, including the body part, the thought, the feeling, and the level of intensity. For example, if you are observing your belly and you feel a twinge of disgust or irritation, write down: "Belly; can't stand the sight of it; feeling disgusted; low-level but ever-present."

Next, move your attention to your breathing. Feel yourself breathing in … and breathing out. In … and out…. Shift your attention to the flow of air coming into your body and imagine it filling up your entire body – both the parts you're OK with on some level, and the parts you might not be so happy with. Feel the air flowing equally to *every* part of you. Notice any feelings or thoughts that arise as you do this, and again, write down any that seem particularly significant.

Next, become aware of your heart-center. If you can, feel the beating of your heart. Keep your awareness focused within your heart-center for a couple of deep breaths. Feel, or imagine, the pumping of blood that is happening as you breathe, without you having to think about it. This amazing organ has been beating for you your whole life long. Take some time right now to be grateful for its tireless service to you. Write down any thoughts that arise.

Next take a moment to do another observational inventory of your body. Has anything changed? Can you feel more of your body than you could before? Do you notice any new aspect of your body that you hadn't noticed when you started this chapter? Are there any additional thoughts or feelings showing up that weren't there before? Simply take note, capturing any significant items that come up, and resist the temptation to label, analyze, or judge any of it.

Hopefully, within the few minutes it's taken you to do this exercise (if you did indeed play along), you have come to find that the simple act of bringing attention to your body results in some real benefit to you. It may have brought more breath and oxygen to your cells, or perhaps your muscles ended up feeling more relaxed, or your inner emotional state got noticeably calmer. Or maybe more inner agitation was brought up – within your mind or within a body part. Whatever the experience, the gift of this exercise is your increased awareness of yourself, and a list of observations that will come in handy as you're looking for the clues that can help you solve the crime of your dieting and weight-loss woes.

Even though this was a simple exercise, which you may have already done a thousand times in your life, the purpose of doing it here was to give you a reminder of how powerful of an impact even the simplest exercise can have when it is done with your neutral, focused *attention*. Let this serve as a reminder to you that looking within, with simple awareness and attention, without needing to change anything, *can* and *does* effect a real change in your body and in your experience of life. And it doesn't have to take very much time out of your day to get you there.

We are setting the foundation here for the work and play you will be doing shortly as you explore how best to heal your dramas and pain-points as they relate to food, your body, and your addictions. The exercises and tools I'll be sharing with you are going to rely on you tapping into your innate wisdom, which contains the natural impulse of your being, which is to move in the direction of self-healing. Sometimes the underlying rules-for-safety mentioned previously cover up this natural impulse, and those are the times you might find you make eating or movement choices that are not in your best interest, or in the interest of your body's natural impulse toward self-healing. Fear not! You'll be discovering exactly why that is, and exactly how to remove those barriers so that your natural impulses can re-emerge.

You've already been introduced to some of these obstacles that can stand in the way of your best intentions and efforts to lose weight, get in shape, exercise, and eat more healthily: food addictions, stress hormones, and a lack of sleep. Another not-so-minor influence, which you'll get to explore in a lot more detail shortly, are the hidden addictions that you, and all of us, have to overcome anytime we want to change a pattern in our lives to something better (different) for us – especially if that something better for us lies smack dab in the middle of the realm *outside* of our known comfort zone.

Even though you're not at all alone in this dynamic of getting tripped up, derailed, waylaid, ambushed, and otherwise thrown into tizzies with regard to all things dieting and weight-loss related, I'm confident that you *do* have the power to step outside of these "habitual behaviors" and become the master of your own actions. Have no fear, the ENLIGHTEN Process will soon help to get you there.

The path you are being invited to walk upon is a path of deep healing. This path will help get you back in control of your eating, stabilize your weight, and tame the inner dialogues that have been keeping you in stress and making choices that no longer serve you. You are going to be uncovering the true influencers of your experiences to date, which up until now have been outside of your awareness because it wasn't yet time for you to see them. This process is fun and very *enlightening*. Are you ready for the ride?

OK. Step 1: Engage Your Inner Witness

This step sounds simple, but trust me – without this step, you will not be giving yourself the true attention and focus that's needed to get to the bottom of *your* weight-loss issues. You are a unique individual, and hundreds of thousands of experiences have happened to you in a different way than they've happened to anyone else. This means that to find your own keys to unlocking your weight-loss story, there is only going to be one place to go that will truly make a difference, and that is *within*.

A really good way to do this is to take a moment, close your eyes, and consciously take three deep breaths. Again, this sounds like such a simple act, but it is a powerful one that will be very helpful to you throughout this journey, and your entire life. It's especially helpful any time you are shifting from one activity into another activity throughout your day – e.g. from working intently to starting to eat your lunch; from eating your breakfast to getting in the car to drive to work.

Here's how it works. You are going to practice this technique of taking three full, deep breaths as you stop one activity and before you start the next one. Simply take a moment to notice that you're going into a new activity, pause, and take three full, deep breaths; then step consciously into your new activity. You may find this simple act alone, when practiced regularly, can begin to help you to change habits and ingrained patterns that otherwise have been kicking in when you simply rush throughout your day from one activity directly into another.

You can try it now by going from the mentally focused state of reading, to this task of pausing, breathing, and observing. Take a moment to stop and take three conscious, deep breaths, and then notice your body. Just that. When you're done with that, come back to the book, taking three breaths again, before continuing reading. How did your body and mind feel before and after taking those breaths? You might find it very helpful to remember this exercise and to do it any time you begin eating, so you will automatically be more present to yourself and your body as you are putting food into it.

A follow-on tip here which may be helpful for you is to do this exercise any time you find yourself frustrated by an eating choice you've made, or you experience yourself having a negative thought about your weight; or you feel abusive self-criticisms attacking you about a part of your body or about yourself. Simply stop, tell your mind you'll get back to it in a bit, and enjoy three full, glorious breaths. After the breaths, feel free to then return to your thoughts, or to follow whatever impulse arises within your newly oxygenated being. Just that. Three conscious breaths.

Once you've become more centered with your breaths, the next step of this process of "looking within" is for you to take a small amount of time to write down a summary of a negative body or weight-loss scene or thought that is frustrating you – that you'd like to put a stop to. You're going to do this as if you are telling it to your best friend. Here are some examples:

- "I can't believe I just ate that container of ice cream! I was doing so well all week!"
- "Why can't I lose this belly fat? All day long, any time I feel my belly, it's a constant irritation to me. It reminds me how fat and lazy I've gotten."
- "I looked at Susan today and noticed her toned belly, arms, and legs and found myself judging her for looking so good. That immediately turned into me judging myself – both for not being able to look like her, *and* for my judgment of her!"

You're going to pick just *one* of the likely hundreds of self-criticizing thoughts or beliefs that pop up for you in your day around your weight or your diet. It's important to pick just *one* thought or scenario to focus on at a time, otherwise the process can get diluted and have less of an impact on your ability to gain new insights into the mystery of your weight-loss whodunit.

So take another moment now, close your eyes, and take three deep and conscious breaths. Then allow *one* of your weight pain-points or your weight-loss struggles or thoughts to bubble up into your awareness. You might try asking your Inner Weight-Loss Guru or guide to help show you the one most appropriate one for you to work with at this time. Allow some time for any one of the following to pop up for you:

Words in your head; an image; a sensation in your body; an irritation; or an emotional response.

When you have one, notice if the one that popped into your awareness surprises you. Is it one that occurs often? Or is it one that you didn't expect was "that big of a deal"? All of these questions are going to help you build up the set of clues that is going to help you unlock the mysteries of your weight-loss story going forward.

In "tuning in" to yourself in this Engage Your Inner Witness step, here are some other questions for you to consider: Are there places and times in your life as you look back on it, where you can now see that you "tuned out" to yourself and to your joys? How often over your years of living within your human bodysuit have your judgment and the conditions you've placed on it being the right size been more important to you than enjoying the journey it was taking you on?

Every time you've had a thought about your body not being good enough, pretty enough, healthy enough, "right" enough, who is it that you thought would care or judge you for it – besides yourself? Another way to think about this question is to answer this question first: If you lived on a desert island, would your weight, your body size, or your body shape matter to you in the same way it does now? If it wouldn't, why not? The answer to this question will show you who you are living for. For whom or for which people do you think your weight issue really matters?

Whatever your answer, know that it is absolutely fine. All of this is simply giving you more information that will be helpful for you as you continue this trip down the rabbit hole within. So much of our life, we are living to please someone other than ourselves. Very often this started as one of our parents. And most often, this dynamic is not consciously known to us – it will surface only once we have the ability to tune in, ask the right questions, and, with curiosity, observe the answers that arise.

We'll be exploring all of these types of thinking later within the process to see how they can be used to help you in your quest to gain control over your eating and your life. For now, I wanted to simply give you some food for thought – which is the kind of food that just might be healthy for us to start getting addicted to!

Note that another portion of Step 1 asks you to look within with *curious eyes*. Curiosity is the opposite of looking within with a "concerted effort in order to figure myself out and beat myself into making a change." Curiosity is one of the characteristics of children – questioning, innocent, and exploratory. It is also the main trait of a character within you I'm going to call your Inner Innocent, who you will be inviting to come out to help you later as you progress further along your ENLIGHTEN journey.

For now, the focus of Step 1 is to turn your focus from a thought or scenario that feels like it has a *hold* over you, into one that you are willing to simply look at, describe, and be compassionate with as you look at it, as you would be if it were a friend sharing it with you. Without this step, we could easily feel the old, familiar, negative, attacking thoughts – or the dieting frustrations – as big scary monsters with thousands of tentacles; and if we do that, it's going to be unlikely we'll want to spend much time with them.

The invitation here is for you to turn within and to look this "monster" in the eye. From the work I've done with hundreds of clients over the last 15 years, I can say with confidence that without fail, every time, the monster has always turned out to be a trick of the light – a wily trick of your Inner Guard Dog. When you can instead look within, with new eyes – with curious eyes instead of fearful, judgmental eyes – then the apparitions can much more easily reveal themselves to be something much more tender and much more in need of your love and attention than your swords and flame-throwers.

It will take courage on your part, the first few times you do this process, to turn within and look with curious eyes at a portion of yourself that you have held as a lifelong enemy or demon. I promise you, though, when you do find the strength, the courage, and the precious time to do this, you will be rewarded with riches beyond your wildest dreams from the beautiful castle that the demon has been trying to keep you from living in.

Chapter 3
Inner Detective

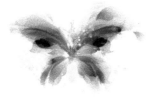

"The universe is not outside of you. Look inside
yourself; everything that you want, you already are."

– RUMI

Learning to Become Your Own
Inner Detective

Step 2: Name the Real Problem/Issue

Step 3: Look at Your Issue and Give It Your Full Attention

Now that you've slowed down, tuned within so you could better sense your body, and taken an initial inventory of one or two sticking points in your thoughts around your body and weight, it's now time to learn how to become your very own best Inner Detective – for real, so you can look at the meanings and clues that lie *behind* all of the daily surface clues you normally see. It's time to get to the heart of the matter, despite all of the tricks that the players in your weight-loss saga have been playing on you to date.

You may have noticed I've been using a lot of imagery in this book so far to talk about the various concepts and exercises I've been introducing. This hasn't been by accident. It's not just a silly whim or writing style of mine that's worked its way into this book. I am using imagery because it is the language of both your intuition, and what I am calling your Inner Innocent. While these two characters are both very different to each other, I've discovered the best way to work with each of them, and most importantly to *speak* with them, is to engage your imagination. Imagination – Image-nation – is a nation full of treasures (gifts of insight and guidance) that all humans can visit at any time. In order to gain access to its treasures, you have to first learn the languages that are spoken there. The national language of Image-Nation is … You guessed it! *Imagination!* The secondary language spoken there is *imagery*.

Why would we want to visit our Image-Nation more often? Well, because it is home to not only our Inner Health Guru, but also our *Intuition* – that magical Oracle that is ever-ready to help us see, and *feel*, what is really going on inside of us in the situations of our lives we feel we need to get better clarity on. Things like: "Why, when I know it's going to make me crash, do I keep grabbing that brownie at breaks instead of drinking some water?"

Whether you feel you are a very intuitive person, or not, you'll be able to use the techniques in this book to your advantage if you simply start utilizing the language of images and imagery more. For instance, if I say to look at the above statement with the eyes of your Inner Detective, it will be helpful for you to picture your favorite detective in as much detail as possible. My favorite detective is Columbo from the long-running TV series of the same name, and I can see him tapping his pockets as if he forgot something, as he hones in on the clues the others think he hasn't seen. For you, it will be helpful to pull up an actual image of your favorite detective inside of you so you can see him or her running around looking for clues – particularly in order to find out who or what your inner saboteur might be.

So try it now. When I say "Inner Detective," what image pops up for you? Is it a fictional detective you have seen or read about? Is it an amalgam of different detectives from whodunit shows? Is it you, with a Sherlock Holmes hat on, with a little dog at your side, looking through a magnifying glass for clues? Is it Hercule Poirot or perhaps Nancy Drew? Any and all of these images can be useful.

Now, if no image just "pops up" for you, that's not a problem. You can either just make one up; or you can think about a beloved detective of yours you've seen on TV, in a movie, or read about in a book; or you can type "best detectives of all time" into Google to see if that jogs your memory (and then simply use one of those images that "pops up" in your search results).

You might be thinking: "What the heck does any of this have to do with helping me get to the heart of my weight-loss issues?" That's probably what I would be thinking, as well, if I were reading this book for the first time. Please bear with me, as I've seen that this type of imagery- and imagination-work does have *a lot* to do with making it easier to light up new understandings inside of you. This in turn will gift you with new perspectives to problems that up until now you may have thought you had explored from *every angle*, yet still haven't been able to solve.

Also, the more fun you have with this exercise of completely picturing your Inner Detective, the more easily you are going to be able to work with him or her when you need to, not only within this process of getting to the heart of your weight-loss issues, but any time you find yourself in conflict somewhere in your life. And the more you work with it, the more you will *want* to work with it, because the more something you're doing is fun, the more you'll want to continue doing it.

If you've now got an image in your mind of your Inner Detective, congratulations! You are now able to communicate more easily with your Intuition and engage its help for the next step of the ENLIGHTEN Process. Your Intuition is your true ally, and it will be taking the form of many of the characters I introduce here, because, well, that's how it communicates with you – through imagery!

Reviewing Step 1, it started with you taking three full breaths and tuning into yourself. Then you were guided to take an inventory of your thoughts and your body feelings and body image issues, and to choose *one* of those issues to work with. If you haven't done all of that, please take a moment right now to do this: breathe, tune in, and then write down one problem area – the one that is currently particularly bothering you.

For Step 2 (Name Your Real Problem/Issue), you are going to ask yourself: "What is bothering me *most* about this issue?" Then you're going to imagine your Inner Detective (or your best friend) is sitting in front of you, as you share your thoughts about the issue. Every time you explain what is bothering you, your best friend/Inner Detective is going to ask you "Why?" or "Why does that bother you?" Here is an example:

Me: Every time I feel my pants tight on my belly, or I look down and see my belly and my belly fat, I'm so irritated with myself and my body.

Best friend: Why does that bother you?

Me: It bothers me because my clothes don't fit as well as they used to and I'm always uncomfortable.

Best friend: And why does that bother you?

Me: Because I have to keep buying bigger and bigger clothes to fit my waist, and now I never look as sharp as I used to because the rest of the pants are baggy on me.

Best friend: So why does that bother you?

Me: Because I want to stay my current size and always look good.

Best friend: Why?

Me: Because I feel ugly, fat, and lazy if I don't look like I should.

Best friend: And why does that bother you?

Me: Because it shows I'm not in control of my eating and I'm weak-willed and a bad person!

Best friend: And why does that bother you?

Me: You're really starting to annoy me! *(Now we know we're getting somewhere!)* It bothers me because I don't want people to see me that way. I'm trying my best and I don't know why I can't stay motivated and eat and exercise the way I should.

Inner Detective: And why does that bother you?

Me: Because I *do* feel out of control and feel hopeless and that I'm going to have to accept that this *is* who I am – a fat, lazy, good-for-nothing human. And what's worse, I feel terrible because this is what I'm passing on to my kids, when I wanted it to be so different for them!

Whoa…. Now that's a different nerve you've hit there that wasn't so obvious with your original statement, "My belly fat bothers me."

This is what you're looking for your Inner Detective to uncover for you. What is *really* bothering you underneath the covers of your surface story? What you are looking for is *any* new awareness that comes. It doesn't have to go this deep. You could easily have stopped with "I'm weak-willed and a bad person!" as your very different pain-point, or at any point along the way where a new angle of your irritation has emerged for you that was different from the surface one.

If you're working through this book doing the exercises as they're described, take a moment now, picture your favorite Inner Detective / Best Friend sitting there with you, and write in your journal what comes up for you as you come under the questioning eye of your Inner Detective. Keep going until you have at least one new take on your irritation than you had before. If you find that what's lying underneath the surface is something you're already consciously aware is a pain-point in your life or your thinking, then this exercise can help you see how it ties itself to other pain-points within you, in order to keep itself in the forefront of your mind, even if you're not consciously thinking of it.

Or it could be that what comes up may be something that is more core to you and which highlights a fear, a negative belief, or an attack on yourself that you had no idea was lurking underneath the surface of your weight or body issue. Either way, the goal of this step is to come more into contact with the core of you – perhaps a more *tender* sore-spot – a pain-point that has been present within you for much more of your life than the surface issue, and one that is more *honestly* what is really irritating you.

This exercise may bring up even *more* irritation or pain in you, but as you read the statement you came to, take some time to really feel into what is coming up for you. That may get you a step below the irritation level, into an emotion that may be even more uncomfortable, like perhaps sadness, shame, or guilt. We will be exploring feelings like these in a later step. For now, simply breathe into it, feeling your body and your feet firmly on the floor, and thank your Inner Detective for helping you get one step closer to solving this aspect of your weight-loss mystery.

It may be tempting at this point to "pull up" from this underlying additional irritation that's been uncovered. I invite you instead to breathe into it, and to apply the same technique you used in Step 1 of the process to simply witness it, without judging it or needing to fix it or change anything about it, the situation, or yourself. This skill you are learning and will be honing throughout this process is going to serve you well, not only in rewriting your weight-story, but also in all aspects of your life. For you to be able to sit with what is coming up for you, like you might do with a best friend, without needing to immediately change it, fix it, or run from it, is in itself a healing salve for your life.

The next step of the process, Step 3: *Look at Your Issue and Give It Your Full Attention,* serves to *anchor* this most bothersome aspect of what's come up for you around your initial irritation. It again may *sound* simple, but it actually can have the most profound effect on your ability to change your weight-loss story.

To illustrate the dynamics of what may happen, imagine a lovely small child coming up to you to share with you something very important to you – like the latest painting she just spent the past hour creating for you for your birthday. She tugs on your pant leg and holds up the painting for you to look at, smiling from ear-to-ear, and so happy to give you this gift from her heart. Imagine now that instead of turning to her, and taking time to look at the painting, and to be with her, you instead just briefly glance at it, say, "That's nice, dear," or worse yet: "Go away, I'm busy!" and then go back to what you were doing. Do you think that is the appropriate and heart-felt response she deserves that would match the energy with which her gift was created for and shared with you?

I know that sometimes things like this happen with the little ones in our care, because we are indeed busy and can't always give everything the attention it might deserve. But with this process, I invite you to give yourself time to make this step work for *you* – to truly turn your attention toward the heart of the situation that arises, and to be with it, giving it your full attention. This is what is really important. You've taken your time to read this far into this book. You've spent countless hours thinking about your food choices, your weight, what you should do next to get it all under control. And now you've gone through these exercises and the steps of tuning into yourself in a new way. Do you think it might be worth it now, to see whatever comes up for you as being something *very* worthy of your attention?

Sometimes the simple act of turning your *attention* toward a new awareness, an old pain, or an emotion that you've been hoping would *just go away*, can have a magical thousand-fold impact on you as it decreases the negative intensity of it. When you can just tune into it and give it your attention without dismissing it, judging it, or reading anything else into it, it can lose its unconscious hold over you with one simple: "I see you!"

Try it now. Look at your irritation – the thing that is *most* bothering you from Step 2. Breathe into it, and then simply say: "I see you." Keeping the tuned-in senses you worked with in Step 1 open, notice what you now feel. Notice how your body responds. Notice what you notice. Give yourself and this problem your *full attention*.

This alone can be the key to truly enlighten your life from the inside out. What you are doing is shining a light of awareness onto something you either haven't looked at within yourself for a while (or ever), or onto something you've never quite seen in this light before. You are checking into your own inner emotional "ICU" (I see you!) with this simple, non-judging attention, and it is oftentimes the first step that's needed before deeper healing can occur.

Getting back to imagery, there are a couple of other images that always come to mind for me when I do this process for myself, or when I am working with others to help them see the new areas within themselves that have been lurking in their shadows, but tripping them up. The first has to do with the concept and imagery of shadows – those apparitions that appear when one shines a light at a certain angle on something that is very often different in size and stature to the size of the shadow.

Often times when we hear the word "shadow," particularly as it relates to the psychological connotation of the term, the image it conjures up in most people's minds is of some dark, scary place within us – some hidden and unknown place that holds our darkest and dirtiest secrets. Oftentimes, we think there are these parts of ourselves we have cast "into the shadows" for a very good reason – because they are things we should never, ever look at within ourselves – our deepest and darkest secrets, which no one (including ourselves) should ever find out about us.

To me, that imagery limits our ability to make use of the deep healing that can come from looking at these "shadows," since it makes us do an about-face any time we even catch a glimpse of one of them, right when the shadow *could* be (and likely *is*) holding up for us the loveliest of painted-from-the-heart birthday gifts, to move us forward in our life's journey!

What we can do if we look toward what is coming up for us is kind of like being given the opportunity as adults to revisit the places that used to be scary to us as children. In revisiting those places now as the grown adults we have become, we have the opportunity to determine *anew* if the thing we had been afraid of doing or being is indeed dangerous for us now, or not. Think of a child, for instance, who sees a scary monster getting cast as a shadow upon his bedroom wall at night when the light of the hallway hits one of his toy soldiers just right. To him, that monster is real – it's there, it's scary, and he is convinced that if he just stays clear of it, all will be well.

But you, as his caregiver, know that the child actually needs to be able get a good night's sleep in that room, so it isn't serving him to be afraid of going into it. In order to help him, you would likely want to help him learn about the nature of shadows – to help show him how it is the shining of the light onto something in his room (his toy soldier) that is casting the shadow he thinks is a monster. You want him to be able to learn how he can play with the light in his room so that he can see that when the light shines differently, it brings a new and different perspective to the room, and the "monster" goes away.

This imagery is going to be very helpful for you to keep in mind as you continue along these steps of your ENLIGHTEN

Process. This analogy is going to come in handy over and over again as you start to uncover thoughts, memories, beliefs about yourself, or habitual patterns that may in the moment look to you like big scary monsters or dragons or big blocks. I will continue to remind you that all of these things may simply be tricks of the light – or tricks of your Inner Guard Dog's light – that have made these things continue to look scary to you to keep you from making changes outside of your old known comfort zone. It's exactly at those "scariest of times" when I will invite you to continue to shine the light of your inner, non-judgmental awareness on them so that you can determine for yourself *now* if they still indicate a dangerous path for you, or not.

Typically, these scary "shadow monster" patterns and negative beliefs come out in full force in our lives at exactly the right timing for us to see that *this old way of being no longer serves us*. When you can learn to pause, take a deep breath, and look for the light switch that can bring you a new perspective on what this scary monster might really be, only then can deep and true healing happen within your psyche. Only by welcoming these otherwise irritating little shadow pieces of yourself in, with this new understanding that they are there to try to grab your attention so you can see how you've been tricked up to now, can you make the changes in your life you are now wanting to make. In this way, you will be honoring these shadows as the beautiful gifts they are – by giving them your simple and full attention.

We don't know what we don't know about these old "demons," only because at some point in our childhoods, if we had lived our lives from whatever positive perspective we now are wishing for ourselves, it would have been unsafe for us *within the context of our environment and surroundings at the time.* This is why they have been cast into the shadows. And because they are the places within us that have gone unexamined, we have continued to remain stuck in a restricted sense of what is and isn't safe for us *despite our more logical current understanding and desire to behave differently as adults.*

Rainer Maria Rilke wrote in his book *Letters to a Young Poet:* "*Perhaps all the dragons in our lives are princesses who are only waiting to see us act, just once, with beauty and courage. Perhaps everything that frightens us is, in its deepest essence, something helpless that wants our love.*"

In this book, and within the ENLIGHTEN Process, you are going to use this concept of your hidden irritations being the *helpless within you that wants your love* to more consciously take a (safe!) peek beneath your surface stories to *gently* coax out your princesses-in-dragon's-clothing. They only need you to simply see them for what they are in order to offer you their gifts. Approaching this process with this kind of awareness, looking at your past dragons through the eyes of love, with simple non-judgmental attention, will be the quickest way for you to shine a new light on your stuck habitual patterns so you will no longer stay stuck in them.

These gems have so much they can teach you. They can show you not only where you've been, but also clarify for you exactly why and how you have been stuck in old patterns and have found it so hard to make the changes you know you'd like to make that would now be healthy for you. If these new behaviors are ones that would have gone against your inner "rules for safety" (ways of being you had to cast into the shadows as your "dragons"), it makes sense from this perspective why you wouldn't have even considered adopting them in your life up to this point. Who would knowingly adopt a scary dragon to live with them?

That means these first steps to unraveling the mystery of your weight-loss woes are the most powerful ones. In Step 1, you get to identify *one* problem related to your weight or your body or a part of body, so as to not overwhelm yourself. You then get to meet and work with your Inner Detective to help you uncover what deeper dragon may be lurking underneath the surface story that simply wants to be seen now. This is Step 2. And your only task in Step 3 is to sit with the new awareness, story, or "demon" that arises – and then give it your full attention. You can think of these steps as the beginning steps of re-writing your weight-loss story. First you have to see the story that you have been writing in order to see why the story hasn't been able to change despite your *wanting* it to change. Only then will you have the whole picture, which is what you need to see so you can effect change going forward.

You can think of the initial steps of this process as simply watching with curious eyes as your past life story unfolds to you in a new way – the way a curious child might look upon a story she's being told at bedtime – curious and expectant to see where the story is going. The simple steps that take you there are:

- Step 1: Engage Your Inner Witness – Look Within with Curious Eyes
- Step 2: Name the Real Problem / Issue
- Step 3: Look at Your Issue and Give It Your *Full Attention*

Case Study

Susan came to me frustrated that even though she had been gaining a healthier attitude toward her food, her eating patterns, and her life, she was constantly aware of her extra belly fat, day in and day out. She realized that all throughout the day, whenever she would see her belly or feel it being touched or brushed up against (from her pants, the seat belt in the car, the purse she was carrying, etc.), she would get extremely irritated, uncomfortable, and frustrated. She assumed this was because it brought up her anger with herself for not having been able control her eating the year before, so the weight she'd lost had all came back, and ended up where it always does, around her belly. Working with her using the ENLIGHTEN Process, I had her first look upon this scenario/situation with curious eyes – to simply see this as an event happening to her, as if it were happening to a friend. She could now use this event to find out something new about her life. This simple change of focus helped her to become more fully present for the next step. I then walked her through the process of doing the inner detective work to root out the deeper reasons for her irritation beyond the ones she could already consciously see. What came out of that was: Yes, a big part of the irritation came from her frustration with herself around her past eating behaviors, but she was already used to that feeling of anger and disgust with herself. Underneath that, what surfaced was much more visceral, and much more painful. It was the thought: "I'm screwing up my kid! I wanted to be a better mom to him. I didn't want him to have to go through life with the pain of being overweight like I did – and I blew it!" With this new awareness, a deep, deep sadness arose within her – a more tender and honest emotion than what she had felt with just her more surface thoughts. And even though the wound that was getting exposed within her was more painful than her surface thoughts, her energy in that moment became more grounded, more honest, and more real. Only then was she in the right place to continue the process, as you will see in the next chapter.

Chapter 4
Feel to Heal

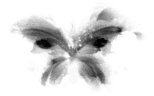

"Your task is not to seek for love, but merely
to seek and find all the barriers within yourself
that you have built against it."

– RUMI

Feeling Your Feelings to Shift Your Energy

Step 4: Ignite Inner Empathy – Honor Your Feeling and
Emotional Bodies

You may now find yourself in a familiar place, heading
toward the same cliff you may have found yourself already
approaching dozens, or likely even hundreds, of times in
the past: "Yes, I *know* I have these hidden issues and not-
so-hidden feelings and negative self-talk with myself, but I
keep...*<insert your favorite repeating pattern here>!"*

With the help of your Inner Detective, you've now
uncovered a sticking-point or problem that the heroine of
your weight-loss story (once again) is experiencing as a giant

weight tied to her waist, which is about to drag her back down into the caverns of out-of-control eating and frustration that she may have just recently climbed out of.

Despite your best efforts, at some point along the journey, *something* happens to trip you up and keep you from reaching your goal of finally being able to find the best way of eating for you, to maintain a healthy relationship to food and to your body, and to pass that victory on to your children. From your explorations in the first chapters, you may now come to recognize this as one of those scary inner demons casting his mighty shadow. This is a trick of your Inner Guard Dog who just wants to keep you safe by keeping you from making any changes in your life which will take you out of your comfort zone and your learned rules about who you are and who you have to be in the world.

In order to proceed along your journey onto a path that is going to bring you to a different outcome, you're going to have to do something radically different to what you have been doing – something radically different to your habituated behaviors at this point along your journey. This is because your habits are your Inner Guard Dog's favorite trick to make his job easy. As long as you kick into a habit that was put into place to keep you from making any changes to your life, you'll be safe from the dreaded world that lies outside of your known comfort zone, and your Inner Guard Dog can go back to snoozing.

Now that you consciously want to step into a *new* pattern, in order to get off of the repeating cycle of letting this negative pattern get the best of you, you may be asking: "Just what courage and energy am I going to have to muster to make this change?" – because you've already tried so much and you're exhausted, right? I know. The good news is that with this step in the process, you are actually going to *free up* a lot of your energy – and in a big way – which is going to make all the difference in the world to you.

This step is one that is likely radically different to what you're used to, not because its content is any different to what you've likely heard and tried to work with before, but because it requires a shift in the *quality of your behavior* – particularly toward yourself and toward your desire and drive to get to your goal of freedom from the weight-loss monsters that have been plaguing you for so long.

To gain a new perspective on what's at play with this repeating pattern coming up for you, you're going to have to start by anchoring yourself within the power of Step 3, giving the one problem you uncovered all of your attention, without judging it. This alone may be difficult to do, so you may want to call on your Inner Weight-Loss Guru and your Inner Detective again, using whatever imagery works best for you, so they can be your guides as you go.

Once you're in that new space with your issue – let's say it's: "I'm so fat and ugly – no one, including me, can ever love me while I'm this way," or some other lie like that. You're going to give that one statement and issue your full attention, without judging it or thinking about all of the additional thoughts that come up around it. You're going to just sit with this *one* problem. From there, with this next step, you're going to then lean even further into it, to *feel* what it would feel like if it were the only true thing about you – the only thing that was grabbing your attention.

You're going to role-play here and you're going to act as if this statement is a fact. You're going to assume it's "who you are" and it's the "truth" of you that's here to stay. (This part likely won't be difficult for you, because this is the lie you've probably already come to believe about yourself.) You're going to feel, and honor, the emotion that really feeling this statement as a truth brings up. With Step 4, you are going to *Ignite Inner Empathy and Honor Your Feeling and Emotional Bodies*. What you're being asked to do here is to switch your focus from your thoughts, to your *feelings and bodily sensations*. You're going to take the leap into the one place you've likely not wanted to go – into the *feeling* aspect of the pain of this painful belief.

To do this, you're going to take three conscious breaths, and afterward, pause. Then you're going to re-read your problem sentence. It may help to say the problem sentence out loud, to let your being know you're ready to do something new here. Then you are going to wait, and listen, as if someone you love and respect is about to impart words of wisdom to you. As you do this, if thoughts come up around the statement, honor those thoughts, and let them know you'll get back to them later. Tell your mind, "Thank you for the input. I'll explore that thought with you later. Right now, I'm going to give my attention to my feelings and to my body."

After you honor every thought in this way, bring your breath and your attention back to your *emotional body* and your *physical body*, asking them to give you feedback. What feelings and which emotions are arising within you as you sit with this problem statement? Where in your body is your attention drawn? Breathe into the body areas that draw your attention to them. Stay focused on your breath, filling in and simply being within these areas that are asking for your attention.

Next label the emotion or emotions associated with the feelings and bodily sensations you are witnessing. Continue breathing, repeating the statement like a mantra, and letting further bodily sensations and associated emotions arise.

Here is an example, with me walking through this process with the above thought, "I am fat and ugly and no one will love me if I can't change that about myself." I feel my solar plexus and I feel resistance to the thought. I feel agitated and irritated – I am resisting going into the thought fully. I notice a new sensation arising now in the pit of my stomach. I'm sensing a lot of fear now. It feels like maybe fear of being cast out; fear of being found out; fear of never being able to change myself. Breathing, I allow the fear to be there – I imagine a scared child in front of me – I acknowledge that she's afraid, and I hold her, telling her: "Yes, I know … I know this is scary."

With another breath, and continuing to repeat the negative statement, I'm now feeling my chest – my heart area. I'm sensing a deep sadness around the feeling that I'm not lovable just as I am. As I feel that, and soften into it, I feel tears coming. I breathe again and honor the sadness, letting it wash over me, as if I were sitting with my best friend who just told me how sad she is. Breathing, crying, repeating the mantra of the negative belief – I'm feeling fully how much sadness I've lived with my whole life, carrying around this belief.

From Susan's story above, as she worked with this step, a deep sadness washed over her, and she realized her "body acceptance issue" was really profound sadness at having failed to protect her child in the way she envisioned for him. This meant that her belly fat irritation wasn't solely a weight issue or an eating issue for her, but rather a constant reminder to her of "being a bad mom" and of "being a failure." Trying to hold back all of the deep sadness these statements brought up, and pretending it wasn't there, had been such hard work that when she was finally able to allow, honor, and really feel the feeling of her deep sadness, she relaxed and became more centered, calm, and present. Even though it seemed like it would be too painful for her to bear, as her tears streamed down her face, she was releasing years and years of tension that her belly weight had been helping her hold onto.

The goal here, and the new skill you will be developing with this step, is to gently *allow* what comes up without needing to change it, fix it, understand it, or make it better. The goal is to be gentle with yourself and the tender feelings that arise; to allow, to witness, and to *sit with* the emotions and feelings and sensations as they come up for you. This requires honing an age-old super-power that all human beings have, but which seems to go dormant in most of us over the course of our lives from living in a society where doing more; being more; getting better; and improving and pushing ourselves, live with us as our gods. This super-power is simple and sweet, and one we have to learn to welcome back into our lives: *gentleness*. Gentleness leads to presence, and presence leads to empathy – which leads in the end to acceptance.

If you find this exercise difficult, or if it's hard for you to sit with what comes up for you without getting drawn too far down the rabbit hole, simply breathe and back out of it for a bit. These are feelings and emotions that you have likely been pushing into the shadows for many years, in order to "just get on with life," so it may feel like if you go ahead and open the floodgates, you're going to be overwhelmed by the rush of feeling, and the fear can arise that it will be too painful. You might also play with calling into your mind's eye the most loving and compassionate friend you can think of, and imagine he or she is sitting with you going through this exercise with you, helping you to breathe and honor whatever is coming up for you without judgment.

I promise you, that if you give your feelings your direct and loving attention, they will not overwhelm you. In working with so many clients over the years through the uncovering of some of the very deeply painful moments in their lives with huge anger or mega-sadness, I've seen that the tension and pressure of *holding these feelings back* and keeping them at bay was *way* more intense and painful for them than what they felt when they were guided to simply *be* with their honest emotions and *feel* them.

These emotions have been trying to get your attention for a while now. When you can simply give them your full attention, they won't have to knock as loudly or bring you as much pain. Think of the imagery of a volcano that has no vent or outlet to let out heat or streams of lava a little at a time. When the pressure builds, that mountaintop is going to *blow* right off! If vents or openings are available, however, the volcano can release the pressure and the heat as it comes, which results in lava flows that gently roll into the sea and turn into fresh, new land.

So again, doing the work of Step 4 to "Ignite Inner Empathy and Honor Your Feeling and Emotional Bodies" may sound simple enough, and like a step you might consider just skimming over so you can quickly move on to the next step. I challenge you, however, to *not* do this, but to instead spend time getting to the *heart* of the authentic feeling that is lurking underneath your surface irritations and frustrations. When you can do this, a profound and impactful *energy shift* will literally occur within you, which has the potential of altering the course of not only your weight-loss saga forever, but also the path of your entire life.

You've likely heard the expression that *what you resist, persists*. In the context of this step of honoring your authentic emotion, it applies here as well. If you spend the majority of your time, consciously (or more likely, unconsciously), pushing past your true feelings, trying to cover up the deep pain within you with another piece of chocolate cake, distracting yourself with staying busy or going shopping, your psyche will say, "That's OK. We'll be here ready to keep popping up for you until you do have the time to be with the truth of you. Take your time."

You see, just like your body has an impulse toward healing, your psyche also has a healing impulse – which is to get your awareness turned toward the light of inner clarity – taking the steps necessary to get you to see the bits of yourself that (for your safety at the time) had been cast into the shadows. It brings up the next places it knows you are now strong enough and adult enough to handle, so you can finally bring them into the healing light of your consciousness to re-assess and determine if they are now safe for you to embody. An example of this is with your tender emotions, as seen within this step of the ENLIGHTEN Your Life process.

If you don't give *yourself* the sweetness of honoring all of the tender places within you that are crying out for your attention, is it any wonder that you so often stand in front of the cupboard looking for something healthy to eat, but instead end up with a sugary treat? Something has to bring you the sweetness that you deserve and crave, as we all do, and if it's not coming from within, then it has to come from "out there."

Again, there is a very real addictive quality to refined sugars and even artificial sweeteners. However, there is also the concept that addictions appear to help fill in holes in our psyches where we aren't feeling a sense of connection with the world around us. In deeply doing the inner work, as you've been doing so far in this process, and simply connecting with your own body and emotions, and sitting with them, you are effectively creating connection for yourself – *within yourself* – in a way that you maybe haven't done since childhood. And this can give you a big enough sense of connection that it can play a huge role in loosening the addictive ties that have been binding you.

Another benefit to honoring your feelings and emotions in this way is that when you go underneath your "protective surface layer" emotions, as I like to call them, you release a *lot* of tension that's been weighing you down not only physically, but also emotionally and energetically. This "protective surface layer" can present itself as the vague sense of being irritated with yourself for not being able to stick to your diet; the harsh negative words you berate yourself with constantly; the moods you experience (and let loose on unsuspecting loved ones) when you feel deprived when you've tried avoiding eating foods you love, etc.

Were you able to feel the difference in your body when you stayed with the more authentic emotions that surfaced as you simply allowed the true pain of your negative belief or thought pattern to be present without needing to fight or change it? For me personally, when I do this, I feel a huge release of tension from my neck and shoulders and have a sense of dropping down into my body and feeling my belly more – often being able to breathe more deeply. I notice with it a huge sense of relief, as well – that I can stop running from what I thought would be the worst demon ever for me to have to encounter: my tender, painful emotions.

You may find it easier to give yourself this gift of being able to uncover, sit with, and honor your emotions in this way with a facilitator or trusted friend at your side. If you don't have those available, you can also use your re-emerging skill of imagination and imagery to call up your Inner Weight-Loss Guru as a trusted friend to sit with you and remind you it's OK to have and to honor the feelings you're having.

Each time you can do this, as you work through this process over time with other negative thought patterns that emerge for you, you are literally lightening your bodily and energetic stress load. This in turn lessens your cortisol levels, which play a key role in your body wanting to increase your fat stores. You'll also find you have more energy to follow through on plans that used to get missed out of sheer tiredness. And with this greater sense of connection to yourself, you'll also be more present in general in life, which can give you a deeper connection to others in your life, by getting you out of the way of your own never-ending thought-stressors. This in turn then reduces one of the factors that play into your food addictions, as well.

You are shedding light into your life, one step at a time.

Please notice that the heart of this step relies on a skill set and a way of being that often goes against the grain of our learned and habitual way of being and existing in the world. As such, it may meet with great resistance from your Inner Guard Dog, whose job it is to keep you from ever going against those inner "rules for safety" that were set up to keep you safe in the world of giants you saw around you at the young age in which you adopted them.

In this case, I am talking about the beliefs that are common to our culture – our universal, cultural beliefs – such as: "I have to work hard to make changes in my life; if something is easy to do, it must not be worth doing; no pain, no gain; the harder I push, the better I will get; to make it in the world, I have to keep pushing myself," etc.

These are all masculine qualities and beliefs that work for certain areas of our lives. However, they are counter-productive to the heart and feeling aspects of this ENLIGHTEN Process, and any process in our lives where we want to sit with and *be* tenderly with a person or child in need. In this case, that person, and that tender child in need, is you and your emotions. Harshness does not serve you in this step – it can hinder you – and likely *has* been hindering you.

Also, most diets and eating plans require a sense of needing will-power: powering through a set of eating plans you've laid out for yourself, staying vigilant and harshly berating yourself if you go astray, etc. I'm here to tell you, as I've seen time and time again, these ways of being are what keep you in a mode of resistance – resistance to yourself and to the more tender areas of your psyche that it's now time for your adult self to see. And since what you resist, persists, this is another factor that has kept you on the hamster wheel of *needing to lose weight* in your life – until now.

Welcome now to the world of a more gentle inner exploration, which will move you toward a new you and an enlightened future.

Chapter 5

Own Your Behaviors

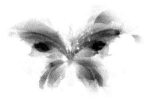

"Yesterday I was clever,
so I wanted to change the world.
Today I am wise, so I am changing myself."

– Rumi

Honestly Owning Your Behaviors without Blame to Take Back Your Power and Tame Your Inner Bully

Step 5: Get Real with Yourself

Step 6: Hold Yourself Accountable

You've now uncovered, below the surface story of your body's extra weight and fat layers, and over the top of any frustrations you've had with your weight issues, at least one deeper issue or negative thought pattern or belief that has been at the root of one of your irritations. This negative thought pattern is a belief you learned about yourself that your Inner Guard Dog has both wanted to make sure you never let the world see, *and* one that you should keep near and dear to you and live by – in order to stay "safe" (i.e., within your learned set of limitations).

That this negative belief about yourself is hidden underneath layers of fat on your body is less of a coincidence and more by design from your Inner Protectress – a.k.a. your loving Inner Guard Dog. Your body can be a helpful ally to the needs of your psyche as it looks for ways to protect you and keep you safe. For instance, if a core belief (a childhood lie) you adopted when you were too little to even be conscious of it, was: "Your body is ugly and something to be ashamed of," then in order to protect you from exposing your body to the world and thereby exposing your ugliness (or your shamefulness), in order to protect that tender core pain and unsafe stance you'd be put into, the body responds to the call-to-action to hide itself – either with skin problems, extra fat, or with dis-eases of multiple varieties.

On top of that potential dynamic, conflicting rules and beliefs got added into your working lexicon of "rules to live by," such as: "To be accepted, I have to have a body that is toned and curvy, in just the right proportions." Never mind that the "right proportions" are open to interpretation. Your conscious mind hears that and says: "OK, that's what I have to go for." Depending on your personality and your inner dynamics, this may be something easy for you to do, so you push past the deeper inner core rule that is saying: "Um, sorry – you have to actually keep yourself covered in fat to protect yourself from a fate worse than 'not being accepted.'" This would mean you might spend a lot of your life "trying to lose weight" to appease your mind and the conscious desire to get healthy and look a certain way, but then no matter what strides you were to make in that direction, if you haven't exposed the deeper pain and more important rule for safety ("You have to keep your body hidden!"), then the deeper rule will win out. Your Inner Guard Dog will see to it that a saboteur of some sort gets inserted at just the right time to get you back to safety.

Hence the repeating cycle of losing weight, only to gain it back again at some point. Until you expose the deeper wound to your conscious mind, and bring it safely into the healing light of your awareness, it will win out every time. You need to examine this deeper wound consciously to determine if it's still something that keeps you safe, or not, because until you do, it will feel to your Inner Guard Dog that letting go of it would be a matter of life and death for you. So what you will be doing throughout this process is coaxing out deeper and deeper wounds – the scary monsters your Inner Guard Dog has been keeping you from looking at – so that you can determine anew if there is indeed still danger lurking within the change you are hoping to make to your body and your life, or not.

The Inner Saboteur (your mind, your thoughts, your cravings) that your Inner Guard Dog can call upon to help with this dynamic is something I call your over-reactive body. Your over-reactive body is made up of a set of e-motions – which can be seen as energies-in-motion. Think of your over-reactive emotions as the ones that draw you in, keep you obsessed and focused on them, and then keep you from being able to be present to yourself or your surroundings (or to the changes you would like to make in your life). They are so amazingly skillful and dramatic, that their acting can keep your attention for weeks, months, and even years at a time without you realizing you've been in the middle of only a grand show. All the while, the actual reality of your life has only been blipping in and out at the outskirts of your awareness. Bravo, E-Motions!

Again, I'm using imagery and analogies here to keep you centered in that part of your being that intuitively understands these dynamics that have been happening to and for you, and to keep your mind active, but not in its usual habitual thinking habit of "Yes, I already know this!" Because – yes, you guessed it – thinking you already know something can be another amazing trick your Inner Guard Dog has used to keep you from changing and moving outside of your comfort zone. This is why I will keep reminding you to keep your curious Inner Innocent at the forefront of your awareness as you go through this process, as that is going to serve you tremendously. She is so curious that she'll never let your mind settle at "OK, yes, I already understand this!" She will keep you curious and thinking about how what you're reading does or doesn't relate to you. She'll have you asking the questions that your Inner Detective needs to be asking to finally get to the bottom of this mystery of why things have been like they have been for you for so long.

OK, so now back to your over-reactive body – that amazing theatre where you have spent so much time as an audience member, and been so drawn into the drama, that you've become a co-participant without even knowing it. The next Steps of the ENLIGHTEN Process are going to get you out of your usual viewing seat, and put you right into the director's chair, where you'll be able to get a clearer picture on the actual *acting* that's been going on in front of you. From there, you'll be able to see if the actions still serve the new story of the life you are consciously wanting to now live.

Practically, what you will be doing in Step 6 is looking at the actions and behaviors that are coming out of your over-reactive body, in order to get a clear and honest view of what *you* have really been doing throughout each of the scenes of your weight-loss saga to date. Keep in mind that the *you* we are talking about is the part of you that has been drawn into the over-reactive body's set of actions, vs. the *you* which might instead, if anchored in your body and in your breath, be able to effectively *respond* to the situations you've been facing.

The word responsibility can be thought of as your *ability to respond* to a situation. In order to respond to a situation healthily and practically, you need to see the situation clearly, be grounded in the reality of the situation, and have a focused and clear mind in order to be able to take the appropriate action fitting for the situation. The state of body and mind you need to be living from in order to respond to a situation is one much like the state you were able to get into with your deep breathing and inner awareness exercise, that brought you to acceptance and attention to your feelings and bodily sensations. Relaxed, open, focused, and alert.

In contrast to this state of being, think about any moment from your past when you can now see you were drawn into the dramas of your over-reactive body. Perhaps a time when your boss berated you in front of your team, or your child purposely ignored you, or your husband didn't listen to you as you were sharing how you felt about an important situation. "How could you be so disrespectful?" Take a moment and step back into that scenario, and observe, with the help of your Inner Detective, your bodily sensations. Is your heart racing? Are you seeing red? Is your breath shallow? Are your muscles tense?

From this place, would you be able to clearly and calmly respond healthily to anything that was before you? Compare this state of your body to the state of your body from the last Chapter and the end of completing Step 4. As you breathed, tuned in to feeling your body, and simply allowed and accepted your true feelings in the moment, even if there was intensity within those feelings, how did your body feel? Was it more relaxed? Were you taking in deeper breaths? Were you calm and focused?

It's going to be important for you going forward to stay aware of these dynamics, and to be mindful that you keep your perspective as coming from the director's chair anytime you are in your over-reactive body theatre. You'll want to stop identifying *as* the actors and simply watch them as they play out the usual weight-loss and sabotaging dramas. Next, you're going to need to explore for yourself whether or not the actions of those actors are ones that are helpful for you (or not) as you continue your work of solving the mystery of your weight-loss dilemmas.

OK, so are you ready? With Step 5, you are going to *tell it like it is* and explore what it is you are *really* doing at the moment one of your repeating habits, negative beliefs, or inner problem areas rears its head. In Steps 2 and 3, you identified *one* core issue, belief, or pain-point that is currently bothering you, you gave it your full attention instead of running from it (the first step in seeing it for what it is), and then you explored how your body felt. By doing this, you could feel what true, deeper feeling/emotion was coming up for you, so you could honor it and start the process of being more fully present to your true self.

In this next step, you are going to take a step back and dive back into your problem statement, taking an honest look at what you are *doing* when you think about and live with that problem statement as your "truth." You're going to look at the behaviors that ensue and determine if they are coming from your responsive body – or from your over-reactive body. Again, all of this is going to be done without judgment. It will be helpful if you imagine you are watching a play unfold that up until now you didn't realize was a play. You had been identified with the characters and didn't have the ability to get the perspective you're going to be able to get to now.

Go back now to your journal and take a look again at your core problem statement. For example, the one that I used in Chapter 3 as an example statement one of my clients uncovered was: "I am a fat, lazy, good-for nothing human!" I'm guessing that yours is also a statement that is not so very nice, and not something you would say to your best friend. Am I right? OK, so imagine now that you are charged with making sure the person who this statement applies to is reminded about this negative "fact" about herself constantly. And not only that, but she should be correcting herself and striving to make herself *not* be that person who is a fat, lazy, good-for-nothing human – so she can finally be "a worthwhile human" in other people's eyes (or she imagines).

If it helps, put yourself up on the stage of your over-reactive body theatre, as the taskmaster/coach of the person who is the fat, lazy, good-for-nothing human who must now be coached on how to change herself for the better. Imagine both the coach and the person being asked to change up on the stage.

Now, look at what this "coach" or taskmaster is saying? How is her posture as it relates to her "underling"? What are the words to describe her behavior? In my client's example, the inner taskmaster is pointing her finger at her "underling" and saying: "How could you let yourself get like this? What's wrong with you? Pick yourself up and get your act together! Why can't you just do what you know you need to do? Why do you always have so many excuses?" And a whole host of other similar bullying statements spews forth. In describing the behavior of this harsh "coach," the words that come to mind for the way she is behaving are: cruel, harsh, demeaning, judgmental, mean, berating, disrespectful, manipulative, dismissive, attacking, aggressive, and vile.

Go ahead now and envision *your* inner taskmaster. Hear and see how she is behaving, what she is doing, and what she is saying. Then in your journal, write out a list of single-word behaviors that describe what you see. Remember, imagine you are sitting in the director's chair watching to see if what's playing out is having the dramatic effect needed for the drama. When you look at the harshness of this behavior and the words that describe it, realize this is how *you* are acting toward yourself anytime one of these underlying frustrations come up for you that you think you already should have figured out or should somehow otherwise "be better at" by now. Can you sense that this negative, bullying energy is the energy you are trying to use to get yourself to make permanent and lasting changes that are "outside your comfort zone"? Can you see why your Inner Innocent may not want to come out to play and step up to the challenges this bullying inner taskmaster is proposing?

The first step to changing this inner dynamic and this intense drama is to *take responsibility* for this behavior that has been spewing forth within you like a load of sludge from the sewer pipe of your past imprinting. It has simply been the response from your over-reactive body, because a pain-point or old wound got exposed. This triggered your Inner Guard Dog to ask the over-reactive body to take over and shut down the "dangerous-to-the-status-quo" change you were trying to make. Perhaps the change was you continuing along your path of taking care of your body and letting it be the healthy slim body you know it can be. Perhaps it was shedding the layer of fat that was protecting the core shameful feelings within you, and you were getting close to doing that, which would have been too dangerously close to disobeying one of your core rules for safety (to hide yourself behind your fat).

It doesn't matter the reason. The goal in this step is to look at what is happening, and to recognize and acknowledge *your role* in keeping this behavior and this meanness going within you as an integral part of your story until now. Perhaps this is a role you didn't fully see you were playing, or maybe one you *kind* of knew you were taking on, but didn't look at with quite this level of detail and scrutiny. Either way, it's time now to see that this *is* the energy you are living out, and it is *against yourself.* Not only is it less than helpful to you, it is downright harmful to the Inner Innocent within you, who wasn't responsible for creating these rules and habits and beliefs she's been having to follow, that she'd learned would keep her safe and keep her old wounds protected.

What matters now is that you see what's been happening. Your over-reactive body has been kicking in at those very moments when you were trying to have will-power, or you needed the energy and presence to make a new eating or exercise choice for yourself. Instead of you having the capacity to *respond* to your life and the situation from a balanced, centered, and productive place, your Inner Bully / Saboteur was called up from the over-reactive body to take you into its dramas, and have you *become* the dramatic evil agent against yourself, in order to keep you from upsetting the status quo that was set up for your safety. In order to step off of this cycle, another act of courage is required of you. It's now time to step back, and to own the fact that the bullying behavior you see *is* indeed behavior that *you* have been acting out against yourself, and it's time for you to *take responsibility* for it – without self-blame.

Again, this is key, because to take responsibility means to give yourself back the ability to respond to your life in a new and healthy way – focused, productive, and in line with the outcome and energy you want to now live your life by. This is an *empowering* step – one that helps you move into a new version of yourself that is present, understanding, compassionate, and kind. It is also a new version of yourself that is, most importantly, *able to respond* to life as it comes before you.

My choice of words in this chapter has been important. Notice that I have *not* said that you *are* any of these things you've been doing. I've framed this whole step in the context of the theatre of your over-reactive body taking over and leading the show when your Inner Guard Dog has directed it to do so, in order to create a distraction any time you've gotten dangerously close to stepping past or beyond one of your outdated rules for safety. That means you have not *consciously* chosen to act this way against yourself. If you were to now *feel bad* about acting this way, or *berate yourself* for being a bad person, then that would *not* be taking responsibility, but rather, once again getting caught up within the over-reactive body's theatrics. Judging yourself also takes you out of responsibility and back into bullying over-reaction. It is simple acknowledgment, without judgment, that is needed.

Taking responsibility for what you *really* have been doing means stepping away from your over-reactive body's dramas, getting clear and more centered, and moving yourself firmly into the director's chair of your own life. It is simply saying: "Wow, yes, this *is* how I've been behaving toward myself," so that you can ground yourself and step out of the out-of-control emotional body and into your core and center. This is the place from which you will be able to live more healthily and free from the dramas the Inner Guard Dog has been using to distract you. This gives you the power to more clearly shine a light on, and heal, the old and outdated lies and rules for living you had adopted that have been tripping you up and no longer serving you.

For Susan, she came to realize as she worked through Steps 5 & 6 that her behavior toward herself, every time she felt "irritated" by her belly fat, had been mean, condemning, and hostile. No wonder she was constantly stressed! After she saw this, she was able to hold herself accountable, without blame, for continuing to carry the story of shame forward in her life as it had become her "comfort zone." She reported back to me about a week later, as she looked back at her days since our work together, that she no longer even noticed her belly fat anymore as things throughout the day touched it. And as she reflected on that, she also realized she had less stress around her eating, and she had much more energy throughout her day. In retrospect, she was amazed at how much energy that "small little irritation" had been taking from her, and how it disappeared overnight when she saw it and then took responsibility for her mean self-bullying behavior that had been bringing her stress!

Chapter 6
Be Kind

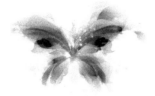

"Raise your words, not voice. It is rain that grows flowers, not thunder."

– RUMI

Re-Parenting Your Innocent Inner Child – Choosing *Kindness* Over Domination

Step 7: Take Your Inner Innocent into Your Loving Arms

With that last step, from this place of acknowledging your own true behaviors, thoughts, and actions that have been at the heart of keeping your weight-loss dramas going, you've taken the reins back into your own hands, and moved yourself firmly back into your own power. Congratulations! This courageous act of consciously and attentively using your Inner Detective to look at the role you've been unconsciously playing in your life story gets you over 50 percent of the way to your goal of stopping the self-sabotaging behaviors that have been keeping you from being free of "needing to diet."

What is needed to get you all the way across the finish line? What you'll need to do next is to dive even more deeply into your being and your heart. This step may require you to develop, or to build back up, a vital yet often underused skill: practicing loving self-kindness. This is often the most difficult task for people, maybe precisely because it requires an infinitely more gentle approach to "changing yourself" than you're used to.

For clues to understanding why this might be such a difficult step for most people, we only have to look at some of the core universal beliefs that most of our families and our culture hold. We have rules telling us: "It's not worthwhile if you don't work hard at it. No pain no gain! You have to work hard in order to succeed in life. Life is hard. You are not enough as you are – you have to keep bettering yourself.... Success is hard work!"

To see where you stand on the spectrum of exploring your own relationship to inner gentleness vs. harshness, all you have to do is take a look at which inner beliefs and/or rules for living you've heard throughout your life regarding easy vs. hard; gentle vs. pushy; self-vigilant vs. allowing; strong-willed vs. trusting, etc. Take a moment right now to journal some of the rules or "statements of fact" you've heard around each of the following. Write down at least five statements for each:

- Money,
- Success,
- Being a good person,

- Getting ahead in life,
- Being an adult.

If you're anything like me, and the vast majority of the clients I've coached, you probably have hundreds of "rules" floating around inside of you that point to life having to be a struggle; or you having to keep yourself working hard to get what you want. If you do have these rules, your Inner Guard Dog will likely work to convince you that this next step in the process is "too simple" to truly be effective; too simple to give you the power I'm going to suggest it will give you to effect real change in your life and your weight-loss sagas.

Step 7 is: *Take and hold your Inner Innocent in your arms.* It sounds easy enough, but remember: your Inner Bully has been the taskmaster that your Inner Guard Dog has been using to *keep* you from thinking you are alright as you are, and that any part of you deserves to be held in a loving embrace. It's going to push back on the idea that your actions are good and right, since they are not within the bounds of the limiting beliefs that have been keeping you within your comfort zone.

When in this step you are guided to look to the "innocence" within you, simply recognize that at first you may have a hard time feeling the innocent you, as that "you" may indeed have "broken the rules" or done something she "shouldn't have done" – which proves she's not deserving. But you are now armed with the awareness of your adult self, and the bright light of your awareness that has been shining a new light on this dynamic within you.

Even so, your Inner Guard Dog will try to remind you that you have not been enough, or have not done enough, or have not been strong enough, or have not had willpower enough, or have not worked hard enough to deserve a kind embrace. And as you've seen from the last two steps, your Inner Bully will therefore be asked to rise up and beat your inner "bad self" back down.

So the imagery that is going to be helpful for you now, to help you to step outside of this cycle, is going to be to call up a younger version of yourself. This younger you should be young enough that it would be hard to see this "you" as being anything but innocent. In that way, you'll be able to see whether or not she truly deserves the treatment your Inner Bully has been dishing out to her. Specifically, you will ask if the harsh, bullying behavior is helping her be able to actually change her habits and patterns or not. I assure you, the energy of this "younger you" Innocent Self is very real. It's a very tender, very important, and very powerful part of yourself.

In order to get in touch with her, you're going to close your eyes and conjure up an image of yourself as a small (very young) child. First take three deep and conscious breaths to center yourself into your heart. Once you're there, ask for an image of yourself as a young child to emerge. Wait and give her time to appear, to get a sense of her, or to hear her. Sit for a while watching her, and then ask and answer the following questions:

How old is this Little You? What is she wearing? What is she doing? Where is she? How does it appear she is feeling (happy, scared, curious, playful)? How is she looking at you (remember that the *you* she will be looking to is the one who represents the actions of the Inner Bully – performing the list of behaviors you listed out in the last step)? Does she trust you? Is she wary of you and your bullying ways? Does she feel safe or scared?

When you have a good feel for her, tune back into your Inner Bully and look again at the behaviors you wrote down from the last step – the stance and actions your Inner Bully took against you to try to fix your problem to date. These actions will be something like mean, belittling, attacking, cruel, heartless, unrelenting, uncaring, etc. Your next task, in your best Inner Bully voice, using your behavior words as your guide, is to take the time to really look at her and to see how this Inner Bully you has been berating her for her transgressions and "wrong-doings." These are the things you think *you* have been doing to create your identified weight-loss problem in your life. In my example, it might sound something like this: "How could you be so stupid and weak? How come you can't control yourself? What's wrong with you? How irresponsible and lazy and good-for-nothing can you be?"

During this time with your Inner Innocent, watch her demeanor and behavior – does it change? How is she feeling now? Really take the time to imagine yourself using all of those harsh negative words you habitually use against yourself to attack and belittle this beautiful, little, innocent one. Watch the scene and *feel* what that feels like. Imagine it, which should be easy since you once were her, and get to know exactly how she is feeling.

For my example, my once playful, happy, and innocently secure little girl is now terrified, shaking, crying, and looking at me in confusion as to why she's being berated so ferociously. Does she deserve this? Of course she doesn't! And neither does *your* Inner Little Innocent!

Until you take this kind of time to look at what these behaviors and your inner thoughts are causing to happen to this tender little you, you will continue this behavior against yourself, thinking it's what you have to do – to follow those rules to "make sure you're working hard enough" so that you finally change "your lazy self!" But your Inner Little Innocent represents the loving heart-space you were born into – she is *you* in your pure genius, before the rules for right and wrong living were imposed on her, before she could possibly have learned to "be bad" and go against you or the rules that she could have no conscious awareness of yet.

Will treating her in this harsh way give you the ability to really help her (as you may have thought)? Will it give you the ability to tap into her energy, her joy, her innocence, and her ability to help you live life from the natural healthy place she knows how to live by – to eat healthily and for the pure joy of it, as all little kids do, naturally? No, it really won't. In fact, it will (and does) do the opposite. Would *you* come out to help someone, or play with someone, or offer your wisdom to someone who was treating you this way? I know I wouldn't!

So again, it's going to feel sad to see how your behaviors have been coming out and attacking your Inner Innocent self, but remember: They have been there as a protective mechanism within you to keep you from "being who you are" – which would be stepping outside of the rules others had imposed on you. What this means is *there is no need to beat yourself up* now *for behaving this way!* It's all part of the once-helpful mechanism that was set up in your inner world to keep you safe as a young child; to keep you from "being too big" or from getting hurt. By looking at things with your adult eyes now, however, you'll be able to see this is no longer a helpful strategy for your adult life.

So the key to shifting your energy is going to be to take time to sit with your Little Inner Innocent and really be with her. Let her know you are sorry – that you *now* see what you have been doing to her – to yourself. That no matter where this fear and concern that she had to be controlled came from, the only one *now* carrying this harsh negative energy and judgment and meanness into your life (that you can do something about) is *you*. And you can hopefully see that it's no longer helpful to you.

Remember that at one point you learned to treat yourself this way in order to be safe. For instance, if you learned it was unsafe to expose your body or your true self, then of course doing whatever you could to "keep yourself down" would have made sense. But now you see that this is no longer what you want – it's no longer what's needed for your safety, nor is it even working to keep you remotely safe or happy! It is no longer healthy for you, or helping you reach your goals of stress-free living around your food choices, your eating patterns, or your exercise habits. This harsh energy and the chasing away of your natural Little Inner Innocent is actually what plays a huge role in *keeping your unhealthy choices* continuing.

So what can you do now to shift your energy and step outside of this negative loop? Quite simply, you can be with her now, and let her know you now see what you (your Inner Bully, as her "protective adult figure") have been doing to her. You were trying to protect her but now you can see how mean and ugly your behavior has been. Feel into what she needs from you now to know it's safe to be with you. Breathe and imagine you have a scared and scarred little child in front of you. What energy do you have to call forth to make her feel safe and happy and free again?

You want her to live freely and happily so you can tap into her energy, which is the pure energy of *you* in your healthiest state. What will it take for you to *now* be with her in a new way? How can you apologize to her and nurture her tender and scared self? What would you say to a three-year-old after realizing you scared the wits out of her and you hadn't realized how much you were yelling at her despite her being completely innocent?

Take as much time as you need to be with her. Continue breathing and feeling into your heart and sensing your body. Breathe and soften your energy. Bring out your most gentle, loving, and nurturing self and energy to calm this stressful scene within you.

In this part of the process, it may be helpful to have a loving friend or a neutral coach guide you through this step, to make sure you are staying out of self-judgment, as that would just be another form of "beating yourself up" which would not be helpful to you now. Remember, the meanness of the Inner Bully was initially put into place from whatever source as a misguided act of love – the strategy you needed at the time to keep you "safe" within the status quo of your environment at the time.

The war is now over. It's time for your Inner Innocent to be allowed out of the bunker that was built up around her to keep her safe from the "world out there" which she learned was dangerous and against which she had to cover herself up, limit her brightness, stay hidden, keep herself down, etc. Take another breath and *feel* the truth of this within your current scenario of having beaten yourself up for whatever "transgression" you thought you'd committed.

Even though the long-held *comfort zone* for your Inner Innocent was to *not* be treated well, to hide, to limit her self-expression, to keep herself down, it's now no longer comfortable, and simply shining the light of your awareness on this fact, now that you're deeply rooted and grounded within your heart, does all the work of shifting that energy now within you.

If you think about how the natural instinct of our body and our psyche is to go toward health, then you can see how going against that instinctual impulse in order to harm yourself, to make unhealthy eating choices, to beat yourself up with your thoughts – these all require *tremendous willpower!* So in those very moments where you have been thinking you've had *no* willpower, it's likely exactly then when your inner (unconscious) willpower kicked in. I would even go so far as to say that the times you are *most* behaving in a way that appears as if you have no willpower (bingeing, over-eating, eating the sugary or fatty treat you said you weren't going to eat, etc.), it's at *that very moment* when your incredible strength and inner willpower to *not* "go toward healing" is strongest. You do not have a willpower problem. You only have a no-longer-relevant-to-your-current-life script "problem."

Now that you have shed healing light on these inner dynamics, and you have re-parented and nurtured your Inner Innocent – in a way that maybe no other adult in your life until now has done – you have energetically shifted yourself at the cellular level. You have changed your "beliefs" in seeing that the old "beliefs" no longer serve you. That alone does all of the work, even though your Inner Guard Dog may right now be growling at you to protest that you are now considering embodying the simple truth of this.

For Susan, this step is what truly brought her into her power and out of the cycle of self-judgment, self-abuse, and the repeating dramas around her fears of failing her son and failing as a mother; around her sense of failure in general. Through this act of kindness toward herself, she was able to finally receive the love and acceptance of herself that she had been waiting to receive from outside of her – from her own mother (who was no longer alive). By seeing how detrimental her behaviors against herself had been, and by apologizing to her Inner Innocent, and holding her in her loving arms, she was able to break out of the habitual cycle her Inner Guard dog had learned she needed for safety. She was also able to clearly see that these behaviors no longer served her in her goal of being a better role model and loving parent to her son. Not only did her relationship to her body, her belly, and her emotions heal through this work, but also her relationship to her son became more stress-free and natural.

Chapter 7
Enlightened Living

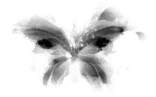

"The universe is not outside of you.
Look inside yourself; everything that you want,
you already are."

– RUMI

Embracing the Rightness of You – Every Day, All Day

Step 8: Embrace the Rightness of *You*

Step 9: Nurture These Understandings into Future Scenarios

If you've been following along and doing these exercises fully, by now you have learned, if even just within the tiniest of baby steps, that by embracing the gentle, nurturing quality of your heart, you have been able to see at least one of your inner weight-loss limiting tales from a different angle and to rewrite the story from your adult perspective. You've been able to re-parent your Inner Innocent, who has been attacked all of these years for something that hasn't been her fault, because of a misunderstanding of the rules your Inner Bully was told you needed to follow in order to safely exist in this world. And you've learned that as a tiny child, you did indeed need to adopt (as far as you learned) these protective stances simply in order to survive your world.

And maybe unbeknownst to you, all of the above realizations have gotten you somewhere between 80-95 percent of the way toward dissolving the impact of those limiting inner tales around one or more of your weight and dieting issues. Even if you've only been reading up until now and not doing any of the exercises, you will have gotten a shift in your energy. If you haven't done the exercises as you go, I encourage you to go back and really let yourself get involved in this deeper way through your active participation. In the end, the good news for you is that if you've gotten this far in the book and understood the concepts and the inner dynamics at play, you have gotten an internal shift of energy that will take you a long way toward your goal of getting off of your endless dieting hamster wheel.

You might be wondering now what the remaining 5-20 percent is that might still need to be addressed? The final stage of the ENLIGHTEN Process is to commit to memory these new awarenesses, inner feelings, and this quality of gentleness within you – in your emotions, your mind, your body, and your spirit. This will help them to be present within you for future scenarios and stories that are for sure going to continue to pop up. You'll see these whenever another "outside-of-your-safety-zone" wish or desire comes up that instinctively would send you back to acting out a limiting habit pattern.

This is the nature of our human journey. I'm here to tell you that you're not alone, and that when you do this inner exploration (and it can even become *fun*, I promise you), your life will change and get lighter in amazing ways – ways you may have intuited before but perhaps not been able to experience fully in all areas of your life.

The future scenarios that could trigger more of your inner limiting and self-abusive stories to arise could be a glance in the mirror; a habitual thought; words from someone outside of you; a stubborn and habitual behavior; or a food addiction. In this chapter, you're going to learn additional tools you'll be able to use when these future scenarios arise so you're not drawn *as* fully downward into the self-hate and self-abusive patterns of your past. This will give you steadier ground to walk on in the time period between the triggering event and the time you will be able to set aside to fully enter into another ENLIGHTEN Process to address the next layer of your unraveling diet-enlightened self.

With this in mind, let's take a step back into the last step – *Taking your Inner Innocent into Your Loving Arms*. Pause right now and take three deep, conscious breaths. After you've done this, engage your imagination again, and call up that beautiful little *you* who you spent time with in Chapter 6, and remember the nurturing energy with which you gave her a true sense of love, acceptance, and safety. Sit with her a while now, and ask her what she would like to do right now. Then simply listen. Follow her joy. Watch how she reacts. See how she feels about herself and how she feels in her environment when she feels safe with you. Watch her as she acts out her joy. Embrace the beauty and the rightness of her. And embrace the beauty and rightness of *you,* as she is simply another aspect of *you.*

Notice your adult "inner observer's" relationship to your Little You. How does your beautiful Little One feel toward you? Does she feel comfortable, safe, and happy? Or does she feel on guard or confused still? Anything that comes up is perfectly fine – you are simply observing her so that you can have an even deeper awareness of your inner dynamics. Notice also how you feel toward her now. What are you feeling when you look at her behaviors and actions? Are you irritated? Amused? Confused? Wanting to change her? Loving watching her? Happy? Content? Again, these are all simply clues that will help you know where you stand with this aspect of your past habitual patterns. You will see if there are still wounded areas that are going to require a bit more of your attention and focus going forward, and if there is now a new sense of calm, self-love, and peace that you can celebrate and come back to for strength.

In reviewing the ENLIGHTEN Process so far, you can see you've done the following:

- Engaged your Inner Witness
- Named your Real Problem and Underlying Issue
- Looked at your problem from all angles and given it your full *attention*

- Ignited Inner Empathy to honor your authentic Feeling
- Gotten real with yourself about your own behavior toward yourself
- Held yourself accountable for those behaviors; and
- Taken your Inner Innocent into the loving arms of your Heart

Hopefully as you have read through this, you were able to feel back into and sense the *gentle* quality this has awakened within you. It's a process of softening to yourself and to your own power. This is the quality of being you need in order to step into your empowered self. Only with empathy and awareness will you be able to step off of the victim-blame-consciousness escalator that you, and we all, ride on so much of our days. There may be a victim inside of you still who is screaming, "Argh! There's nothing I can do about this – I just don't have the willpower or the inner strength to stick to doing what I know I should!" with self-berating and belittling energy, trying to get you to change, or to be shamed into changing.

Or there might be the voice of your inner blamer, saying: "What is *wrong* with me? Why can't I just be strong enough to do what it takes? I have to force myself to go to the gym and to restrict my food intake, but I don't seem to be able to do those things – it takes too much of my energy, and I'm exhausted!" Up until now, both of these voices may have gotten you to some level of success throughout your weight-loss adventures. The problem is that neither of the voices has been loving, kind, empathetic, or gentle, so your inner being eventually rebels under the pressure that either one puts her under. This means that both of these strategies are actually very *dis*empowering to you – they either continuously paint you as the victim (so what can you do?), or they pressure and attack you mercilessly like a drill sergeant (because you know deep down you're bad, lazy, and hopeless if left to your own devices).

In order to step outside of this pattern of shame and inner attacks, you will need to get more and more practiced at getting into this softened and empowered inner state of honest awareness and self-kindness. Only by stepping outside of the old patterns will you truly be able to be served on your quest for a lighter and healthier you. In this way, you will also see benefits in every area of your life, as you take the reigns of your own inner chariot back into your own hands, and become the master of your own destiny.

How you experience the world and all that it brings into your life is completely within your own power when you practice engaging the power of your Inner Detective along with your fabulous Heart to root out the old "demons" which no longer serve you. In this way, you will be able to see them as the nebulous shadows they really are, which are completely not dangerous to you anymore. And then it will be natural for you to hold yourself in a loving embrace, knowing that it wasn't you who consciously chose to believe in these fears and limiting beliefs. You simply were taught them – as a strategy to keep yourself protected and safe in the world that presented itself to you when you were very young.

And until now, it's likely you hadn't yet learned to shine the light of your awareness onto these old stories in quite this way before. Remember now that this journey back home to yourself is a life-long process. It is the process of *unlearning* the "truths" you'd learned about yourself that would have been too dangerous for you to let out into the light of day previously in your young life. This means the beautiful mechanisms of your psyche (your Inner Guard Dog) had simply cast them into your shadowy dungeons in the name of safety for you. It said: "Stay here. Don't venture into the fullness of you. This small subset of ways to live is the only safe place for you." In this way, you came to live within your "limitations" and the "wrongness of you" and your perceived "weaknesses" – as an act of self-preservation and self-love.

Now that you are able to see this – now that you have enough conscious awareness of these dynamics – you can define a new place of true safety for yourself – one of true inner empowerment and of embracing yourself as a loving and loved child of the Universe. And from this more empowered place, you can now employ the work of the final two steps of the process in order to much more powerfully anchor the work you've done so far.

With Step 8, you are going to: *Embrace the Rightness of You*. What do I mean by that? Well, up until now, particularly in the context of the problem around your weight that you were able to identify at the beginning of this process, you had learned to focus on all that is *wrong* with you – on all of those things you had to look at and struggle to figure out how to correct, work on, and *fix* about yourself. That required a lot of energy and willpower you had to always muster in order to *work on and fix* this "broken" part of you.

At this point, however, if you've been following the plotline of all of these inner dynamics that have been at play within you, you'll be able to see that the following is truly what's happened, and none of it points to anything about you being broken:

- The situations in your life, in this case around food and/or weight-loss and weight-gain, had become charged with e-motion, energy-in-motion, within you and your over-reactive body, anytime an old wound or place of perceived danger within you has been triggered – based on past childhood experiences you were not even consciously aware of until now.
- Your Inner Guard Dog has been kicking in, doing his loving duty to protect you from the perceived danger (by calling on your over-reactive body and your Inner Bully to keep you in your comfort zone and safely within your valley of self-limiting behaviors).
- Your over-reactive body has harkened the call and kicked in to ensure that appropriate actions are being taken to "get you back to safety" (via binge-eating, eating something you consciously know or feel isn't good for you, postponing eating better until tomorrow, and then finally, beating yourself up for all of your transgressions).
- Your Inner Guard Dog was then able to rest again, knowing that you're back to the safety zone of your

learned behaviors for safety, so you can just veg out now and hopefully not get up the silly notion to think of "getting back on the wagon" again for a while.

- If you had then at some point used your conscious willpower to get yourself back on the track your conscious mind wanted to take you, then your Inner Bully stepped in to make sure to keep you on this "cycle of 'safety'" by lashing out at you, or berating you for being so weak as to have to keep trying to figure this all out. All of this was done, again, in self-protective "love" to keep you from shifting into a new empowered mindset of change, gentleness, love, and true adult safety – because that would put at risk all of the rules from childhood that are revered and must be followed at all costs (according to the mechanism of your unconscious mind).

- This inner set of emotions and behaviors has been kicking in to keep you safe, and all of this requires tremendous energy, willpower, and inner strength on your part. And because every organism's nature is to self-heal and self-protect, this learned behavior of actively going *against* your nature has been quite an amazing feat that "you" (your inner actors and characters) have been pulling off to perfection all of these years!

- In this context, the "weakest will-powered" moments of your past have been actually pointing to and highlighting the amazingness of you. For you to have been able to follow these unconscious directives has been nothing short of miraculous. And I'm guessing this is likely the opposite view of yourself you've had anytime you've "fallen off the wagon" of some new diet or exercise plan.... Right?

- Until you learned about the power of your Inner Detective being able to shine the healing light of your awareness onto these situations in new ways, you had only been acting out in loving service to your old rules of safety anytime you have engaged in self-sabotage or self-recrimination. It could not have been any other way. Since this is the pattern you learned, unconsciously, to be the best course of action to keep you safe and alive, you *had* to act in these seemingly "self-sabotaging" ways.

Given all of the above, I ask you now: Have you done anything wrong up to now, with the limited perspective you've had (because of the cleverness of your Inner Guard Dog)? Or have you been acting to the best of your ability to keep yourself from perceived dangers you simply didn't know how to re-explore until now? Now is the time to *be gentle with yourself!* It is the only way to move in a direction that is outside of your old habits and patterns.

Back to Step 8: *Embrace the rightness of you.* Remember that the truth of you is not defined by your actions – those have arisen out of a number of various factors, most of which have been hidden from your awareness until now. Who you are is a child of God – you *are* the Innocent One who is below these actions – the one every cell of your being has been trying to protect until now, with love: This was misguided action with loving intent. You have done nothing wrong. This is the journey that awakening to these changes must take within you, and within every human. It is the Hero's Journey. And you *are* the hero of your own journey.

The first step of consciously stepping onto your path of joy and weight freedom is to honor yourself as the hero of your own journey. To take back your power and to observe yourself as often as possible from this new 10,000-foot view – to see and honor the *rightness of you*, right now, just as you are.

Now that you are on this stable footing, the final step of your ENLIGHTEN Process, Step 9, is for you to: *Nurture this gentleness within you in order to carry these understandings into future scenarios.* Like water over time has the power to create deep grooves, and even canyons, within very solid bedrock, the power of your awareness and the inner empathy you will have through these new understandings has the power alone to wash away these old core patterns that had until now been the bedrock of your psyche, and therefore your experiences. Your growing inner gentleness and self-acceptance have the power to effect all of this change for you effortlessly, if you will invest the time, your breaths, your kindness, and your gentleness to return to it over and over again.

Remember always these truths: To keep you safe, the Universe has been giving you exactly what you learned you needed for your safety, as defined by your Inner Guard Dog (psyche). It has been helping you to keep your rules for safety alive, bringing you all of the experiences to maintain your status quo and bring everything you needed for that into your reality and life. For instance, if you learned that to be safe, you had to *hide who you truly are* (because you learned behaving in a certain way would get you punished, for instance), then any time you may have tried to shine or "be you" – the Universe saw to it that the right people, experiences, or circumstances would show up in your life at just the right time make sure you weren't allowed to truly shine, in order to enforce this as a true "rule for safety" for you. Perhaps every time you lost weight, you got unwelcome attention; or every time you tried to eat healthily, and felt a new energy within your being to truly thrive as your full self, you would get the urge to eat something you know isn't healthy to you (which would bring you back into safe "hiding" mode).

The message for you to now carry forward into your future scenarios is that your inner ability to follow these outdated rules, despite your being's inner impulse to always go toward health and healing, is nothing short of miraculous. You are an amazing human being, worth loving, and you are not in any way wrong for living out these patterns. *Be gentle with yourself and keep this view as you encounter future stressful scenarios, and your path forward will be full of joy and much more effortless and empowering than it ever has been before.*

Chapter 8
Supportive Resources

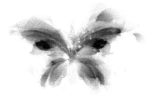

"Your acts of kindness are iridescent wings of divine love, which linger and continue to uplift others long after your sharing."

– Rumi

Resources to Support You with Your Newly Freed-Up Energy to Go Forward in Lightness of Body, Spirit, Mind, and Emotions

Congratulations! You are now well on your way toward dissolving the impacts your inner limiting tales have been having on your body image and on your weight-loss and dieting goals. You will also find that other patterns of your life will be positively affected by the self-awareness work you do around your weight-loss goals, as you'll be uncovering many of the places within you that up until now had not had even the tiniest glimmer of light or love shone upon them. What you will be exposing are all of those parts of you that you thought were unlovable and shameful. The parts you've now come to see (and will continue to see whenever you engage the ENLIGHTEN Process) were your loving, protective strategies to stay safe in whatever scary world your Little You had learned how to survive in.

The good news is you now have a way to empower yourself to re-write the scary monster-shadow stories of your past by looking on them with simple loving attention, awareness, presence, empathy, and kind understanding. And make no mistake about it – doing this work has a powerful positive impact on you at the *cellular level*. In his book *The Biology of Belief,* Bruce Lipton explains it this way: "Beliefs and thoughts alter cells in your body. [...] People need to realize that their thoughts are more primary than their genes, because the environment, which is influenced by our thoughts, controls the genes." So when you get to expose and dissolve these inner negative thoughts and see them for what they are, you are dissolving them at the cellular level into the bright flame of your loving heart.

In this chapter, I'm going to share some additional tools with you, along with some ways of being that I've seen work to bring more of this cell-changing, healing light into your body. You will be using your loving attention to effect positive changes to your mental state, your weight, your eating health, your stress levels, your metabolism, and your overall health. Being able to gain new loving perspectives of yourself and your life, particularly around your dietary habits and eating patterns, is going to go a long way toward helping you live a happy and healthy life in a body that is exactly the right size for you.

As you've experienced so far within the ENLIGHTEN Process, the simple act of looking upon your inner dynamics with loving kindness can be enough to help lift you out of the constant stress and damaging effects of your harsh Inner Bully's berating and abusive energy. That freedom from perpetual stress is one of the key reasons for doing this work, as that alone will have such a profound influence not only on your energy levels and your ability to love yourself, but also on your overall health.

This puts you in the most empowered space to find and utilize other tools that can reduce your inner stress levels and add to these health benefits. One such tool I want to remind you about, from earlier in this book, is one that is simple enough that you can easily use it day-in and day-out to maintain a reduced level of stress. It is something you can easily work into your day any time you are eating. Ideally you will set this up as a simple ritual you are able to start every meal with, because of how quick and easy it is to work in.

You have hopefully already practiced this while reading this book – taking three conscious breaths between stopping one activity and starting another one. This simple ritual is one you can bring to your life any time you are about to eat something. Before you put that first bite of food into your mouth, you can simply pause, close your eyes, and take one to three deep and conscious breaths. When you're done, open your eyes, really look at the new piece of delicious food you are about to eat, and as you take that first bite, give it your full attention. Notice the smell, the taste, the texture, and the nourishing life-giving energy the Universe is blessing you with in the moment with this morsel of food.

Note that by acknowledging the nourishing deliciousness of your food, it brings you into the present moment, and potentially into the space of gratitude, which also brings you into a higher vibration within your body. This acknowledgment of the goodness of the food you are about to eat can be done at any time, for *any* food you are eating – whether it is a piece of chocolate, a piece of fruit, a piece of lettuce, a steak, a doughnut, or a bite of ice cream. *All* food, when eaten with enjoyment, minus the attacking beliefs associated with you telling yourself you shouldn't be eating it, will bring you into the power of gratitude, light, ease, and love in the moment, which in turn will have a powerful positive impact to how your cells respond to your eating *and* to the food you are eating.

It's been my experience that what is as important, if not more so, than *what* you are eating, is the *quality of being* you bring to your experience of eating. How loving, full of gratitude, and stress-free you can be at the very moment you are eating anything will directly determine the health-benefits it will have for your body. The energy you bring to your eating also plays a big role in determining the energy that the food you eat will bring to your body, your psyche, and your life. By practicing this simple act of slowing down, and grounding yourself within yourself with your conscious breaths as you begin to eat, you will be gifting yourself with the full light and energy of the food you are eating, making every food you eat more of a super-food for your cells. Bringing your presence and conscious awareness to what you are putting into your body is a simple yet profound tool you can use to gain mastery over your eating health.

I recommend setting a goal for yourself to do this for three days in a row to start with. Make a conscious decision that every time you switch from a non-eating activity into an eating activity, you will first take 1-3 deep breaths. If you catch yourself chowing down on something and then realize you forgot to take some conscious breaths, don't worry! Beating yourself up is *not* allowed in this practice. Instead, simply notice, and choose at *that* moment instead to take your three conscious breaths. And if you find you've just finished gobbling down your food in a habitual manner at any time throughout the day, without having remembered to consciously breathe, again, no worries. Simply notice that, and then think back on the amazing food you've just eaten, breathing as you do so, and bring all of your love and gratitude to yourself and to the delicious food you just ate.

In his excellent book *The Slow Down Diet*, author Marc David writes: "We need to work less to achieve more. We need to stop fighting food and start embracing it. We need to stop punishing our bodies and start providing for them. We need to slow down and enjoy and then we'll get the results we've been looking for – and sooner than we expect." Simply slowing down and *being with* yourself and your food as you are eating it is key. Notice any thoughts that arise, and notice if your Inner Guard Dog is kicking in. If he or she is, simply take note, and know you can write down any thoughts that come up and set up a time for yourself to work through another ENLIGHTEN Process at some point in the future with those new limiting thoughts you're witnessing. The feelings and thoughts could be about anything – from irritation (with the ritual or with yourself), to boredom, frustration, anger, curiosity, or humor. Simply note the feeling, and breathe into it, knowing there must be a dynamic at play within that you simply haven't yet gained a new perspective on. See your little Inner Innocent within you, and simply acknowledge her, however she is feeling – and breathe. This simple act of loving awareness and kindness towards yourself will go a long way to resetting your stressful eating and self-sabotaging behaviors. *Go easy on yourself!*

Do not underestimate how healing this work is for your body and how much positive impact it will have for you and your weight-loss goals. Turning your inner self- and body-hatred around directly relates to improving your health profoundly from the inside out. A research study published January 26, 2017 in the *Obesity* journal found that fat- and self-shaming (and not obesity itself) is what directly increases a person's risk for metabolic syndrome and its subsequent health issues. Researchers in the study found that participants who internalized stress from weight-related stigma were over 40 percent more likely to have metabolic syndrome than participants who did not internalize that stigma. This finding is significant! The conclusion of the study is that if the stress of being overweight can be reduced, the disease burden on the body will also be reduced. This is why the ENLIGHTEN Process, and other work you do to be present and grateful for your body and your food as you are eating it, is so very important and powerful.

Until you do the inner work to tame your Inner Bully and re-parent your stressed and beaten up Inner Innocent, the belief patterns inside of you that keep telling you how fat, lazy, and worthless you are because of your weight or body shape are taken as "truths" and are the real culprits keeping you unhealthy – *more so* than your food choices or your inner character or make-up. Every time you look lovingly on the old rules-for-safety – instead of thinking there is something wrong with you – you are literally changing your health at the metabolic and cellular levels, which is where the change has to take place for you to succeed at life-long weight and body freedom.

If you also think about where all of these attacks and the fat shaming on our overweight bodies have come from, you will see that the media and our culture play no small role. Our inner image is in constant comparison to the media images of what "health" and "beauty" should be. We're also up against a diet industry whose main job in order to stay in business is to convince us we are not the weight we should be, and we are in need of a product or service they are selling. In creating this book, I had to fight against feeling a bit like I was becoming a part of that industry. In the end, however, I came to see my book instead as a Trojan horse – as a *light* shining out from within the dieting industry world that is going to cast out the shadows that have been alive in too many of us for far too long.

Healing the idea that there is something inherently wrong with us – if we don't look a certain way or can't maintain a certain weight – is what this book, my process, and my work on this planet is about. The very thought that there is something wrong with us, whether it be with our bodies, our weight, how we look, or some other aspect of how we think we must be to please others "out there," is such a big stressor on the body, that *these thoughts alone* are the actual cause of dis-ease and weight-gain in our bodies, keeping us on this downward spiral of related health issues.

Something else that the weight-loss and dieting industry continually bombards us with is the idea that you have to *get control* over yourself, and muster up the willpower, strength, and inner fortitude to perfectly follow this diet plan, or that exercise plan, or ideally as many of their tips that you can at a time! While there is of course something to be said for the positive health benefits that so many of the diet and exercise plans out there can have for us, if we try to follow them before first doing this inner work, we are doomed to fail, because our inner saboteur is going to do its job to make sure we instead stay safely within our comfort zones of learned unconscious rules about who we need to be and what we need to do before it will let us change ourselves into a "new person."

It's important to remember that when something is enjoyable, you will continue doing it. When it is work, and done with the mentality of it being "hard work," it will be the first thing you drop when you get stressed, ill, or tired. When something has to be forced and you see it as hard work that requires willpower to maintain, you won't be able to retain it as a routine in your life, because your soul's impulse is always to go toward joy – the Joy of Being – which is the celebration of life and your inherent right to enjoy your ride on this planet.

While there is something to be said for "tough-love" and boot-camp-type programs to help kick-start you into a new routine of healthier exercising and eating choices, if these are done in a way that simply mirrors the limiting patterns of abuse you're already used to from your Inner Bully, they won't be bringing anything new to you and your weight-loss drama. Instead, they will simply be another powerful way to activate and keep alive the very saboteurs within you that have convinced you this "pushing" and drill-sergeant mentality from outside is what you deserve and need. They will reinforce your childhood wound that you need to "fix your broken self."

There is nothing to fix when you are living a life free from your inner demons and the lies which tell you there is something wrong with you. Your body will naturally go toward health, love, and longevity when it is freed up from the constant stress of inner self-abuse, inner and outer fat-shaming, and the weight of having to *hold up* all of the inner conflicting rules, beliefs, activities, and limitations that have been keeping your Inner Innocent in protection and hiding mode.

It is time to get off of this never-ending fat-shaming cycle, one beautiful body and soul at a time. Working with the ENLIGHTEN Process, slowing down, reframing your relationship with yourself and with the food you are eating, taking one conscious step at a time after another, is the most powerful, simple, loving, and kind path you can follow to take you there.

Chapter 9

The Journey Continues

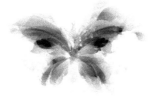

"Yesterday is gone and its tale told.
Today new seeds are growing."

–RUMI

Continuing Your Inner Journey to Enlighten All Areas of Your Life

Some additional supportive systems and tools can also work well in conjunction with the ENLIGHTEN Process to help you bring about a healthier state of mind as you do the playful Inner Detective work to coax out the old patterns that no longer serve you. Some of the tools I have found helpful include daily meditation, Nia (dance/yoga), left-handed journaling, and other forms of body and energy work. These all have powerful and slightly different ways of helping you uncover the inner body- and emotional-energy patterns that have gotten stuck within you from childhood, in the name of self-protection. I'll share more with you on how I've worked with these for myself and with students and clients a little later in this chapter.

Before doing that, however, it is important to first talk about some of the things that can keep these beautiful inner-awareness processes and tools from working, specifically as you go to apply them toward your weight loss goals. It's a very common thing for people I've worked with to be masters at using some or all of these various empowering inner tools, but to still find themselves being repeatedly challenged in finding lasting success with losing their excess weight and keeping it off. I believe a big reason for this comes from the fact that the make-up of the body is directly related to the thoughts we are running. Our thoughts quite literally play a big role in shaping our lives and our bodies in our day-to-day lives. Given that the cells of our bodies are regenerating all of the time, have you ever thought about why our body doesn't create the healthiest and most fit version of itself and its different parts when the old cells slough off and the new ones generate?

It's because the cells get their blueprint for what they are to become from our thoughts and the old patterns already in place, as we have seen earlier. The body and our deepest, innermost beliefs and rules-for-safety always work together as friends. For example, if an unconscious part of yourself holds as a deep core belief that it is dangerous to expose your true self to the world, your body is going to hear that rule, and then work to support that rule – either with extra layers of fat, or for those of us who work hard to "get in shape" as their addictive pattern, with layers and layers of tight muscles.

When this happens, a secondary thought pattern can then kick in to lock those physical patterns in place which are trying to keep us safe: We berate ourselves for what we see in front of us that we don't like. Or we start acting like drill sergeants with ourselves to keep up the intense workouts or pressure on ourselves if we *do* start approaching where we want our weight to be. And, as you've seen throughout this book, since those harsh words, demeaning behaviors, and negative self-talk act as stressors to our bodies, they in turn help keep our "safe" extra weight on us via the stress hormone cortisol. Either that, or they leave us in a constant state of worry about maintaining our "success" once we are at a healthier weight, which also creates stress within the body (and mind).

Because the body is the outward representation of *"who we think we are"* and who we present ourselves to be out in the world, it is easy, and very common, to associate our sense of *self* or *who I am* as the body: "I am my body." As you read this, hopefully you sense that, at a minimum, this sentence is an incomplete representation of *you*. Who you are is much more than your body. You have a mind, and thoughts, and senses, and emotions, and all of them together make up your sense of *you*. There is your personality that also goes along *with* your body to represent who you think of as *you* as well. Take a moment right now to feel this for yourself. Take a full deep breath, and picture yourself standing naked in front of a full-length mirror, looking at your body. Chances are you find yourself to be less than happy with some part of your body, or your shape, or your looks – as so many of us do.

Notice now what thoughts come to you as you are looking at your body. What are you thinking of your body, as you see it in that reflection – when you think of it as *you?* Why are you concerned about the things you think are not perfect or are not how you'd like them to be within this beautiful human-suit vehicle you walk around in? Are you experiencing thoughts and feelings of disappointment, shame, worry, or frustration? Are you thinking about how others will judge you or act toward you with the current state of your body and its shape? All of these things are very normal to feel and sense when you take a good look at your body. One big reason is that our culture associates beauty (and therefore inclusion, love, and worthiness) to your looks and to your body maintaining a particular perfect shape. Note that this image of the "perfect body" is different in cultures all around the world. And still, even though we all can logically mentally understand this, why does it remain so difficult for us to separate our sense of *self* or our sense of *being worthy* from our body shape and size?

Again, it has to do with our deep conditioning. We have learned to see each other's physical bodies as *who they are* before we see that they also are made up of an emotional body, a mental body, a metaphysical body, and a soul. So naturally, as we then learn the rules for how we need to behave and who we have to be to "fit in" and to "stay safe," those also become embedded as rules into our physical bodies. You may have learned a number of rules that were so important to your being at the time you learned them that your psyche pushed them into the unconscious so you could go on automatic-pilot in order to live by them without having to overtax your decision-making brain. This is the healthy mechanism we've already explored – your Inner Guard Dog's super strategy for keeping you safe in the most efficient way.

So now, as you look to uncover which rules might no longer be serving you in your adult life and which may no longer be the conscious desires you have for yourself, particularly around your patterns for keeping weight on or gaining weight back after losing it, it is going to be important to dive deeply into various forms of your belief systems as they relate to your view of yourself in relation to the world around you. Your body is reflective of all of your thoughts, not the least of which are those very thoughts you have no idea you're holding.

In the ShadowPlay work that I do – which is the ENLIGHTEN Process followed by a facilitated deeper dive into a related set of hidden beliefs – my class participants and coaching clients utilize stories and conflicts from all areas of their lives in order to get to the heart of their weight and body-image issues. While the agenda they may be working with is to lose weight and keep it off, the stories we'll explore together are any ones that bring them stress in their daily lives (relationship issues, family issues, money issues, work issues, etc.). This is because there will always be a tie-back into the body and its cellular structures from every outside story or drama being explored. As you work through the ENLIGHTEN Process yourself going forward, keep in mind that it will be helpful to look at any of the troubling thoughts, dramas, or self-attacks you see happening in your life – not just the ones you specifically see as weight issues.

As I said, going through a few sessions of the ShadowPlay work I offer, or doing this type of deep Jungian work in some other way, will go a long way toward getting you a clearer view of the many hidden stories your Inner Guard Dog uses to keep you tied into your limited, but hopefully safe, world. These inner limiting rules around your weight-loss struggles, as well as all of your life struggles, are ones you are not supposed to consciously see, which means they may be tough to see on your own without some outside support. You can begin your journey into this level of deep inner exploration to unravel the layers affecting and limiting your best conscious weight-loss efforts by running through the steps of the ENLIGHTEN Process on a regular basis. I recommend that, at least once a week, you journal about one repeating pattern or thought that has been grabbing your attention throughout that week. You could set up a time in your calendar weekly to do this – maybe as your end-of-week review on a Sunday evening, for example. In addition to working this process to uncover your barriers to self-love, I'll describe in more detail some of the other helpful tools that I have found can be used in conjunction with your journaling with the ENLIGHTEN Process.

The first additional support tool I use on a regular basis in my own life is an hour of meditation every morning. I resisted even the idea of meditation for the longest time in my life, because when I'd hear the word meditation, my mind would conjure up some sort of tortuous, painful experience of having to sit in silence with all of my crazy thoughts making me … well … crazy. Then I discovered that a great way to meditate is simply to sit for any length of time without moving. When I tried doing that for a half hour, letting whatever thoughts came up just be there without getting attached to them, the half-hour flew by in no time, and I realized in that time I'd gotten insights into a problem I hadn't even realized was on my mind. Well now, that was easy!

Thus began my understanding (late in life, but better late than never!) of what a powerful tool daily meditation can be. I invested in the Holosync system of listening to audiotapes that use sound waves to more quickly bring one into into deeper brain wave patterns (see appendix), but you don't have to do anything too fancy to work the benefits of meditation into your life. You can simply wake up a half hour earlier to spend some quiet time without moving, to let your brain rest at a level below your normal waking conscious mind. This will help you grow your self-awareness muscle, which can be of great service to your Intuition and your Inner Detective, helping them more easily be able to solve the mystery of the secret limiting beliefs that have been keeping you stuck in patterns that no longer serve you.

Another powerful tool I've used to help me uncover the real heart of my body issues or weight frustrations over the years is to have a dialogue with a part of my body I'm not able to love fully – by journaling with my non-dominant hand. This is a technique I learned many years ago, and it works nicely as a way to get the creative mind / intuition to uncover beliefs and any negative self-talk your body has been feeling, but that you may not have been aware of. What you'll do, particularly if you are having difficulty coming up with the underlying issue of your current story as you are *Naming the Real Problem* in Step 2 of the ENLIGHTEN Process, is you will use your non-dominant hand to draw an outline of your body, and then highlight the area of your body that is bothering you.

If you notice you are continually stressed and feeling frustrated when you feel or notice your belly fat, for instance, here is a process you can follow. If you are right-handed, use your left hand to draw your body, circling or putting an X on that part of your body that's captured your attention (or your hate or disgust). In this case, it would be your belly area – particularly the fat residing there. You will then ask your belly fat, writing with your right-hand, what message it has for you – what would it like to tell you about why you've been unable to stop noticing it? Switching back to your left (non-dominant) hand, you will then write out an answer, allowing yourself time to sit in silence for a bit to give your left hand the time and freedom with which to write. The reason for this is that it is then coming from a different part of your brain than you're normally used to thinking from. If the answer is unclear or incomplete, you will then use your right hand to ask any clarifying questions. In this way, you will have a dialogue with a deeper part of yourself, which is one way to get insight into these normally hidden-from-you beliefs that often would otherwise only be possible to see with the help of an outside facilitator.

Here is an example of a left-hand journaling session from my past. The left-hand writing is written in italics:

[The left hand drew a body with a lot of scribbles over the belly area, which was drawn wider than the rest of the body.]
What do you have to share with me? How are you feeling?
I don't like you!

Why not?
Because you don't like me or understand me!

I'm sorry. I don't really know you, and I'd like to get to know you. What can you share with me so I might understand you better?
I'm here to protect you!

To protect me from what?
From the world out there.

How are you protecting me?
I'm helping you hide!

Hide from what?
From the people who could hurt you!

Who are those people?
The meanies.

Is there a group in particular who have been the meanies I'm hiding from?
All men.

Really?
Yes.

But I've known a lot of men who haven't been mean at all!
Have you?

Yes. But is that a belief I hold, that men are meanies?
Yes.

So when I'm hating you I'm not honoring the role you've been playing to keep me safe?
Right.

Thank you for being there to protect me!
You are welcome!

What do you need from me?
Love and understanding.

And if I love you, will you reassess with me if "all men are meanies" is still a true statement for us?
Yes.

In this way, I was able to uncover something about my life I hadn't been consciously aware of – that some part of me (a part I don't often give respect to) has been allowing me to hide and protect myself from "all men." This was interesting, because consciously I've always felt safe around men and have always had what I would consider relatively good relationships with the men in my life, without any particularly traumatic or terrible experiences I can think of consciously.

Yet in listening to that layer of love and protection I normally call my "extra fat I have to get rid of," it got me to take a look more deeply at the history of my romantic relationships. When I did that, I noticed a pattern I hadn't noticed before. While I consider my intimate relationships all to have been relatively healthy, I hadn't been able to get any of them to last for more than a few years at a time. And while I had wondered about this, I chalked it up to growth and me and my partner simply growing apart. But with this new information from my belly fat, I could see how I had in subtle ways always hidden the true me from those men, for fear of them not understanding me or loving me if I were to share my true self with them. Because I had learned at some point in my growing years that men are less able to be sensitive to my feelings and emotions – the part that makes me vulnerable (and ultimately that makes me who I am) – I embodied the rule that it would be better to hide my true self, and to not really *be* in relationship with men fully. So after a while of hiding in these ways, no relationship could carry on for a long time, as I'd feel unseen or like my partner just didn't "get" me … because *I* was never fully in any of the relationships to begin with. *A-ha!*

And all of that came to me as a gift through my belly fat! No wonder I hadn't heard the message before. I've spent so much of my life wanting that part of me to just disappear, I couldn't see the message it had been storing for me all of these years. When you learn to soften and look at the irritations in your life through the clear looking glass of enlightened awareness, the parts of yourself and the areas in your relationships that once seemed like your biggest problems can instead become your biggest gifts. This is particularly true once you have the tools and the support to unbury the treasure of their messages.

Another way to call in the creative, intuitive support within you is by engaging in internally focused movement forms, like yoga, Nia, or other forms of dance. Doing so can help you explore the various places within yourself that are calling out to you as the next area for you to work with. When you move with joy, or perform any activity that brings you full-on joy, you are giving your heart and your Inner Innocent just what they need to become open and relaxed. If you do these types of practices right before engaging in an ENLIGHTEN Process or a facilitated ShadowPlay session, you will be able to much more quickly shift into new and more gentle perspectives on your issues, which is where the power of the work comes from.

The same goes for any other creative endeavor you engage in fully, with joy, such as painting, writing, singing, playing the piano, etc. The more time you spend with these activities in your life, the easier you'll find this inner exploration and approach to be, because your intuition and your Inner Detective will become strengthened through these activities, making your process of uncovering your Inner Saboteur and his tricks that much easier.

Chapter 10
Conclusion

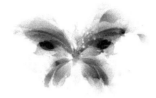

"The wound is the place where the light enters you."

– RUMI

Letting Your Body Lead You Back Home to Loving Self-Kindness

Every part of your body holds the jewels of your deepest memories, thoughts, and habit patterns. Your Inner Guard Dog's job has been to protect these old "treasures" (rules for your safety) using not only your over-reactive emotional body, but also your physical body. Your thoughts, which get stored within your cells, have a direct effect on the shape, size, flexibility, and stability of your body. What this means is that you can look to your body to provide you with the clues you need to shine a light on these old patterns that no longer serve you.

The next time you feel a body part grab your attention – perhaps as something you can't like or accept – take a moment to simply become aware of it from this new perspective that it may have a very important message for you. You can slow down, take three conscious breaths, and look upon that body part with the curious eyes of your Inner Detective. This will help you begin an *enlightened* journey back home to a more authentic you.

When I work with clients over multiple sessions, deeper life understandings very commonly arise from the triggers and traumas of their body and weight issues. In this way, clients get to see that the body and the old, outdated rules for safety are intertwined and influence one another. What's more, it turns out that when a client gains a new awareness that shows a belief to no longer be valid, the body's shape and "energy holding areas" can and do change (like in my case, with my belly fat). This can happen by the client suddenly losing the cravings she'd had before, or suddenly finding she can stick to an exercise or eating plan. The converse is also true. If the client has *not* yet seen how her body is related to the old habitual patterns within her thinking, if she then tries to change a portion of her body with a new exercise or diet plan, her Inner Guard Dog will be on high alert, as the protection mechanism is being altered, and an alert will sound: *this is not safe!* The body can then easily gain back the weight, and gain the upper hand, as it has many more years' experience holding onto these patterns (which come from the inside out) than the person has trying to change herself from the outside in.

The steps of the ENLIGHTEN Process will take you a long way on this journey home to yourself – to honoring yourself in new ways. When you turn inward with your awareness in new loving and gentle ways, only then will you be able to look with new adult eyes on old behaviors and patterns that have been blocking your attempts to lose weight and keep it off (which, in the end, is really about finding happiness and contentment in your life). Having an outside coach, or an "Outer Detective," who can help you see things from a different perspective can speed up the process of finding these hidden beliefs tremendously, because on your own, you are up against that Inner Guard Dog. She knows your every weakness, and has all the best strategies for making sure she gets her way (to protect you from the scary prospect of stepping outside of your "comfort" zone – which is no longer comfortable!).

My talent and passion in life is to help people shine a bright light of new awareness into these areas of hidden, outdated rules for safety, so that the bits of their true full selves that had to go into hiding can be welcomed back home to the open arms of their understanding and accepting heart. I see myself holding a flashlight, like a female version of Columbo, intuitively knowing how and when to shine this light of clarity at just the right angle, at just the right time, to allow those I work with to easily see their next inner "monster" as simply the harmless shadow of an outdated rule it really is.

Remember that the learned "truths" about yourself, which got imprinted into you at a young age, are the real reasons you experience the world exactly as you do. If you are seeing something in your body (or in your world) that you don't like, know that a part of you feels it's exactly what is needed for your safety. If it's something that bothers you, that's good news! You now can look at that irritation as a gift – a gift that is tapping you on the shoulder saying: "There's something to learn here; there's something from your past you're holding onto; it's time to welcome it back home to the light of your loving awareness if it is something that no longer serves you!"

This ENLIGHTEN Process on its own, or combined with the follow-on of ShadowPlay coaching, acts as a kind of conscious soul-retrieval, with the side-benefit of showing you exactly why you've been experiencing life in the way you have been all these years. Your struggles represent where your new conscious desires are coming up against your old rules for safety, such as: "I have to look pretty to be loved as a woman," coming up against "I have to hide my beauty in order to be safe (treated equally, not objectified, loved for who I really am)." By seeing these dynamics with adult eyes, and rooting out the specific rules you learned to keep you safe, you can finally step off of the victim train, get perspective on your past struggles, increase your self-love and empathy, and be empowered to now write the new chapters of your weight-loss story. You will do this by seeing that you didn't choose these ways of acting in the world in the first place, so how could beating yourself up for them be helpful or even make sense? It all comes back to gentleness, and shining the pure light of new awareness onto old stories – which does all the work.

Go gentle. Always gentle. In this way, you will find your way back home to yourself and to a happy, whole, and empowered life, with your Inner Innocent and your Heart leading the way.

Further Reading

- *Bright Line Eating* by Susan Peirce Thompson Ph. D.
- *The Slow Down Diet* by Marc David
- *The Biology of Belief* by Bruce Lipton
- *The Essential Rumi* by Coleman Barks
- Holosync® Meditation Technology:
  http://www.centerpointe.com/

Acknowledgments

The inspiration for this book came while I was on (yet another) fun multi-hour phone call with my amazing and lovely sister, Barbara Dumbrigue. She constantly shows me what courage and inner strength look like as she looks within, cries, faces herself, laughs, grows, and gets up another day to keep at the inner work that has enriched not only her life and her family's lives, but also my life a thousand-fold. Thank you, Barbara, from the bottom of my heart, for always supporting me and for being the best playmate and guiding light for me throughout all my years on this planet.

To my friend and Star Sister, Pam Pedziwiatr – thank you for your unwavering belief in me, and for helping me so many times to get out of my own way so the light within me could shine through. You are a great friend, and I cherish your friendship.

To my friend Alfonso Sosa Cordero – thank you for your love and support over the past few years. Your strength and vibrancy have been an inspiration and beautiful gift to me.

To all of my amazing, lovely, supportive, and fun siblings, nieces, and nephews – thank you all for bringing so much Joy, Love, and Laughter to my life!

To my mischievous, funny, and supportive brother John Evans – you are the yang to my yin, and I thank you for keeping me grounded, productive, on my toes, and laughing.

To my goofy, fun, helpful, and kind-hearted brother Chris Evans – thank you for bringing the laughter and the heart of you into my life – from Big Bird to Dr. Seuss to Sean Stephenson – you always know how to pick the fun ones!

To my lovely sisters-in-law, and sisters-in-spirit, Karen Evans, Patricia Evans, and Michelle Alessandri. Thank you for your beautiful friendship over the years, and for bringing me the gift of three more amazing sisters into my life!

To my amazing niece and nephews, Rose Dumbrigue, William Dumbrigue, and Jack Dumbrigue – thank you for teaching me what unconditional love is, and for completing my heart.

To my hundreds of students, who have trusted me over the course of many years to hold space for them as they uncovered and lived out their courage, tenacity, and their inner empathy through thousands of hours in the hot seat, as detectives, and as loving inner-nurturers – thank you! Your presence in my life has blessed me more than you know.

To all of my teachers and mentors whose teachings and presence have played a big role in helping me uncover and strengthen my gifts of insight, intuition and light energy healing – particularly John and Esther Veltheim, Robin Rice, Sharon and Trevor Hart, Sean Stephenson and Mindie Kniss.

To all of my loving friends who have supported me in my journey toward the Light of Living – with special call-outs to Gudrun Lentner, Sylvia West, Kai Christiansen, Kelly Atkins, and Debbie Moran. Thank you for the fun, the playfulness, and the belief you have always had in me. I am grateful for your beautiful hearts and presence in my life.

To the Morgan James Publishing team: Special thanks to David Hancock, CEO & Founder for believing in me and my message. To my Author Relations Manager, Tiffany Gibson, thanks for making the process seamless and easy. Many more thanks to everyone else, but especially Jim Howard, Bethany Marshall, and Nickcole Watkins.

And for you, Mom and Dad, without whom I wouldn't have picked up my tenacity, my spark, my creativity, my humor, my playful spirit, and my sense that life is more magical than it might first appear. I hope wherever you are, you can feel the love and the light in this book that are a direct tribute to your beautiful selves.

About the Author

Linda Evans is the founder of the Sonoran Light Healing Center and an international speaker, seminar leader, light-worker, and self-awareness coach. For the past 15 years, she has helped hundreds of people get to the heart of their core body, weight, and relationship issues, and back to living life as their most ideal, happy, and vibrantly healthy selves. Her deeply insightful and healing work is a combination of heart-based energy healing, Jungian depth psychology, and light-hearted play and imagery.

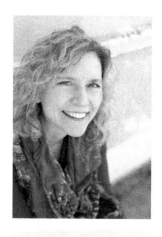

Linda was put on the planet to help change humanity's focus from a mindset of limitations, blame, and victimhood to one of empowerment, clarity, and self-love. It is her mission to get as many people to join her on this journey back home to their True Selves, not only because the time is ripe, but also because the trip is a whole lot of *fun!*

Linda now lives among the saguaros of the beautiful and healing Sonoran Desert, and holds local retreats and private immersion sessions in addition to her global weekend seminars and online coaching sessions. She finds the energy of the desert to be magical and a helpful partner in the light-healing work she does to help clients return to the vibrant health and boundless Joy that is their birthright.

For rejuvenation of her soul and spirit, Linda finds time to sing in a women's acapella chorus, dances, plays golf, and spends as much time laughing with those most dear to her as she can.

Website: www.theenlightenprocess.com
Email: linda@theenlightenprocess.com
Facebook: www.facebook.com/EnlightenYour
LifeWithLinda

Thank You

I hope reading *Enlightened Weight Loss* was both an enlightening and deeply healing experience for you. You have now stepped onto a path of deeper empathy and compassion for yourself. Should you find future moments in your life where you come up against old eating and weight demons, may the tools from this book help you look upon them with new, understanding eyes.

I sincerely hope this book leaves you with a deeper sense of your own internal power that will assist you in rewriting the stories of your dieting (and your whole) life that no longer serve you. This work and inner discovery is a life-long process, and a journey worth taking.

To help you deepen your understanding of the ENLIGHTEN Process, so you can more easily put its steps into practical action in your day-to-day life, I've created a 3-part e-course as a companion to this book and my gift to you. In it, you'll find even more helpful tips, examples, and case studies I wasn't able to include in the book. You can get access to the videos here: http://www.theenlightenprocess.com/